Also by Elizabeth Plourde, Ph.D.

Your Guide to Hysterectomy, Ovary Removal, & Hormone Replacement: What ALL Women Need to Know

Hysterectomy? The Best or Worst Thing that Ever Happened to Me? A Collection of Women's Personal Experiences

Available from New Voice Publications at:

www.nvpub.net
www.store.newvoice.net

Sunscreens – Biohazard

Treat as Hazardous Waste

Elizabeth Plourde, Ph.D.

Printed in the United States of America

Plourde, Elizabeth
Sunscreens – Biohazard: Treat as Hazardous Waste

| ISBN: | 978-0966173558-1 |
| LCCN: | 2011906150 |

| Cover design: | Marcus Plourde, Ph.D. |

Published by:	New Voice Publications
	P.O. Box 14133
	Irvine, CA 92623

Dedication

This book is dedicated to our planet Earth and to all the life forms living on it, whose health and survival are dependent upon its being safe and pure — free of toxins that cause harm.

♥ *Elizabeth Plourde, Ph.D.*

Acknowledgements

I would like to acknowledge all the researchers who provided the material for this book. I thank them for being willing to document their findings regarding the damage caused by the chemicals, which we as consumers have taken for granted to be safe. The world owes all of you a debt of gratitude.

♥ *Elizabeth Plourde, Ph.D.*

Table of Contents

List of Tables and Figures

Tables

Figures

List of Abbreviations

	Description	Solar Spectrum Wavelength Range		
IR	Infrared radiation wavelengths			
IRA	Infrared A radiation wavelengths	700	– 1,400	nm
IRB	Infrared B radiation wavelengths	1,400	– 3,000	nm
IRC	Infrared C radiation wavelengths	3,000 nm	– 1 mm	

IU   International Units

mcg   microgram
µg/L   micrograms/liter
mm   millimeter
ng/mL nanograms/milliliter
nmol/L nanomoles/liter
nm   nanometer

TiO_2 Titanium dioxide

UV	Ultraviolet radiation wavelengths			
UVA	Ultraviolet A radiation wavelengths	100	– 280	nm
UVB	Ultraviolet B radiation wavelengths	280	– 315	nm
UVC	Ultraviolet C radiation wavelengths	315	– 400	nm

ZnO   Zinc oxide

Preface

While spending time in Hawaii in the summer of 2010, I saw headlines in their newspaper saying "Coral Reefs Dying due to Global Warming". This did not make sense to me as I have been swimming in Hawaiian waters for over 40 years and this year was the first summer that I had to coax myself into the water, one inch at a time, because it was so cool. I have been a medical researcher and author of health books for 20 years and decided to start investigating why the coral would die; it certainly was not due to warmer water temperatures. When I immediately uncovered an article that unequivocally demonstrated that coral die just from exposure to sunscreen chemicals, I knew I had write a book to start warning the world that sunscreens were jeopardizing the beautiful coral reefs of the world. It is not only coral, it is the whole marine habitat that is threatened as many fish and species of marine life depend on the coral.

I had no idea at the time that I would uncover the importance of the biochemistry training that I experienced to become a California licensed Clinical Laboratory Scientist, as well as my 20 years of being a medical researcher on hormones and hormone balancing.

As I uncovered the impact these sunscreens are having not only on coral, but fish and birds as well, I began to be horrified at how life on the earth is being threatened. Then when I found studies that showed these sunscreens chemicals are in the blood of almost 100% of Americans, including the ones who state they have never used a sunscreen, I realized if fish and birds are being reproductively impacted, then humans exposed to these chemicals must be too. Our babies could start exhibiting some of the same problems that scientists are discovering in most all of the life forms they are testing with sunscreen exposure.

I also had no concept at the ubiquitousness and pervasiveness of so many products on the market today that now have sunscreen chemicals in addition to those dedicated as sunscreens. In fact, it is almost impossible to find products without them.

I became even more dedicated to this work when I realized that vitamin D deficiency diseases, all but wiped out a century ago, have been returning due to the encouraged behavior to shield against sunshine. The body needs the sun's rays in order to manufacture its essential vitamin D within the skin.

Thank you for caring enough to pick up this book. Please care enough about the planet and your family and friends to get multiple copies and pass them on to as many people as possible. If we stop buying products with sunscreen chemicals, they will stop making them.

Thank you for sharing the journey of protecting our home, the planet Earth, and protecting your families and friends,

♥ *Elizabeth Plourde, Ph.D.*

Sunscreens – Biohazard

Treat as Hazardous Waste

Part 1 – The Sun's Rays and Sunscreens

Chapter 1
Sunscreens

Introduction

We are warned that sunlight is our enemy and causes skin cancers and the potentially deadly melanoma. In support of sunscreen use, the U.S. Centers for Disease Control and Prevention (CDC) updated their Website guidelines August 10, 2010 stating:

"Slather yourself in sunscreen. The sun emits three types of ultraviolet radiation, conveniently named A, B, and C. UVC is not generally a concern. A good sunscreen will block UVA and UVB. Wear sunscreen with a minimum of SPF 15. SPF refers to the amount of time you will be protected from a burn. An SPF of 15 will allow a person to stay out in the sun 15 times longer than they normally would be able to stay without burning. The SPF rating applies to skin reddening and protection against UVB exposure. It does not indicate any level of protection against UVA. A good broad-spectrum sunscreen will contain additional ingredients to block UVA, such as Mexoryl, Parsol 1789, titanium dioxide, zinc oxide, or avobenzone."[1]

This urging by the government and the medical community has indeed been overwhelmingly responded to by the public. Around the world, hundreds of millions of dollars are now spent each year to protect our skin from the sun's rays. In the U.S. alone, between 2002 and 2009, sales for sunscreens grew from $100 million to $798 million.[2]

Yet, does the course of action they are telling us to take really provide us with what we need to know to protect ourselves, our families, and the planet? Is staying in the sun longer, because we no longer show signs of burning, good for our skin? Are these chemicals really safe to place on our skin? Are these chemicals safe for the planet's waters that we swim in, need to drink, and essential-to-life for the fish that live in them?

This book will answer these questions by looking at what the scientific and medical studies have been and continue to reveal regarding sunscreens and their affect on the biology of all life forms.

Sunscreen History

Egyptians utilized certain plants to protect themselves from the sun, although we can assume they did not know how or why they worked. Modern science has identified what they used were the chemicals gamma oryzanol and jasmine. The gamma oryzanol is an antioxidant that is still extracted from rice bran today. It protects the skin from solar radiation damage because is absorbs UV radiation. Jasmine works because it mends skin damage by healing DNA at the cellular level in the skin.[3]

Over the centuries, humans have devised various ways to protect their skin. The Greek Olympic athletes utilized mixtures of sand and oil to protect their skin while training for their events. Christopher Columbus wrote that the Caribbean islanders painted their bodies with reds, blacks, and other colors as a form of sun protection for their skin.

In more recent history, the first commercial ultraviolet sunscreen became available in 1928. This was the chemical para-aminobenzoic acid (PABA), which the manufacturers marketed for filtering out what are called the UVB rays from the solar spectrum. Efforts to utilize chemicals other than PABA have been sought as there are many shortcomings in using PABA. In addition to skin irritation and allergic reactions, it discolors fabrics. Also, being water-soluble, it is not as effective in water or under sweaty conditions.[4]

As the awareness of the sun's potential for causing skin damage was realized, many sunscreen formulations began to hit the market, and in the early 1970s, the Sun Protective Factor (SPF) labeling that describes the amount of time a person could stay in the sun due to blockage of UVB waves was introduced to the U.S.[5] It was at this time that improvements to PABA were made by creating modified forms (PABA esters) that made it less allergenic and less soluble in water, so it did not wash off as easily. However, a common derivative of PABA (para-aminoazobenzene) still induces allergies in approximately 16% of the population.[6]

Research articles published in the 1970s and into the early 1980s showed the use of PABA led to an increase in cell death as well as DNA damage, and by the late 1980s concern began to surface that PABA could be potentially carcinogenic.[7] In 1993, a study identified that PABA in the ester of padimate O, even though harmless in the dark, upon exposure to sunlight becomes capable of causing mutations in DNA, which could result in cancer.[8] As different researchers came up with conflicting results, no definitive conclusions were drawn at the time, however, PABA esters gradually became less common as ingredients in sunscreens.[9]

In the 1970s, studies began to appear recognizing that, in addition to the UVB radiation damage to the skin that the SPF sunscreens were designed to stop, UVA radiation also created damage, and these solar rays went deeper into the dermal layer of the skin.[10] With researchers confirming that damaging solar radiation was not just from the UVB range, but also from the UVA range, Europe approved a UVA filtering chemical in the 1970s.[11]

In the U.S., it was not until 1988 that the FDA approved a sunscreen with UVA filtering abilities. The U.S. CDC is now recommending that the sunscreen you use has to block UVA as well as UVB radiation, however, over the years the public has been unaware of this. As a result, people utilizing sunscreens have been staying out in the sun longer than they normally would have before the advent of sunscreen use, while feeling assured that they are protecting not only themselves, but their children as well, from developing skin cancers.

The Skin Sunscreens Are Trying to Protect

Skin Anatomy

The skin is divided into three main layers. They are the:

Epidermis: outer layer

Dermis: middle layer

Hypodermis (subcutis, or subcutaneous): inner layer

These layers and their cells are shown in Figure 1.

Layers of the Skin

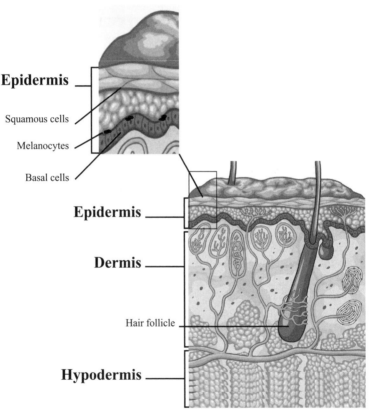

Figure 1. Epidermis (with squamous cells, basal cells, and melanocytes), dermis, and hypodermis.

The outer epidermis layer is divided into 5 layers and contains the three cell types:

Squamous cells: flat, scaly cells in the surface.

Basal cells: round cells underneath the squamous cells.

Melanocytes: produce the melanin that gives skin its color.

These are the cells that give rise to skin cancers and melanomas:

Squamous cells: squamous cell carcinoma.

Basal cells: basal cell carcinoma.

Melanocytes: melanoma.

The dermis layer contains the sweat glands and hair follicles, as well as the collagen that helps the skin stay young looking, while the hypodermis contains the fat producing cells.[12]

Chapter 2
Skin Cancers

Do Sunscreens Protect You From Skin Cancers?
If using sunscreens works to prevent skin cancer, then the incidence of skin cancers would go down with the advent of sunscreening agents and their mass utilization. What are the facts about skin cancers over the time period since sun filtering chemicals have been introduced and promoted? Let us look at whether sunscreens have reduced the incidence of skin cancers that they were brought onto the market to do.

Melanoma
Melanoma is a cancerous growth of the melanocytes, which are the cells responsible for the production of the brown tanning pigment, melanin. Melanin production is the protective reaction of the skin in response to the sun's radiation.[13] Melanin is capable of absorbing solar energy and dissipating it as heat. However, it can only absorb so much, and when it is overwhelmed, the chemicals that are created can lead to cellular damage and cancer.[14]

Some studies show the incidence of melanoma has increased, while others show there has been a decrease in its incidence over the last 30 years. In attempts to analyze these conflicting studies, researchers utilize a tool called a meta-analysis, where they combine all similar studies and submit the data to a statistical analysis to determine if, collectively, they show a trend. With studies showing both increases and decreases in melanoma, mathematically the collective analysis produced findings that indicate there has been a negligible impact on melanoma since sunscreen use began.

As a result of the studies canceling each other out, we have to let the melanoma statistics regarding its incidence rate speak for themselves. In looking at statistics from governmental agencies, the World Health Organization (WHO), and well controlled studies on the actual numbers of cases of melanoma, there has been a tremendous and consistent rise in the incidence of melanoma cases.[15] The incidence rate of melanoma has risen dramatically over the last 30 years, which is the period of time that sunscreen use has been widely publicized to be used generously by everyone.[16]

In 1973, the U.S. incidence rates among White males was 6.7 per 100,000, and among White females 5.9 per 100,000.[17] Since that time, the rate has steadily increased, so much so, that 35 years later in 2008 the rate for men had increased more than five times with 34.1 per 100,000 and increased nearly 4 times for woman with 23.1 per 100,000. Whites are much more susceptible to melanoma as shown by the incidence rate for Blacks in the U.S. over this same time period is approximately 1 per 100,000. The 2008 incidence rate for Blacks with both sexes combined was 1.2 per 100,000.[18] These figures are displayed in Table 1 below.

Table 1.   **Melanoma – U.S. Incidence Rates**

				(per 100,000)
	1973	1985	1995	2008
White:				
Males	6.7	17.2	23.5	34.1
Females	5.9	12.7	16.4	23.1
Males / females combined				27.6
Black:				
Males / females combined				1.2

Throughout the 1970s and 1980s in the U.S., melanoma incidence rates increased faster than any other cancer. The trend continued through the 1990s as the U.S. Surveillance, Epidemiology, and End Results (SEER) statistics for the years from 1973 to 1997 continued to show that malignant melanoma was the most rapidly increasing malignancy in both sexes.[19] In 1999, melanoma was the 6th most common cancer for U.S. men of all races. By 2004, the combined incidence rate for U.S. men of all races increasing to 22.9 per 100,000 made melanoma rise to being the 5th most common cancer among men, while it became the 7th most common among females.[20] This increase in melanoma becomes significant when looking at the lifetime risk of an American developing melanoma in 1935 was only 1 in 1,500 individuals, when by 2007 this statistic had climbed dramatically to 1 in 52 individuals.[21]

Incidence Rates: All Cancer Types

During the years 1992 and 2008, the U.S. incidence for all cancer types in White males and females combined declined 9.2%. Over these same years, the melanoma incidence rate in White males and females combined rose from 17.2 per 100,000 to 27.6 per 100,000; an increase of 60.5%.[22] A study published in 2005 in the *Journal of Clinical Oncology* looking at those in the under 20 age group concluded that between 1973 and 2001 the incidence of melanoma increased rapidly among children. The incidence increased exponentially in White children after the age of 10, with a much greater increase in females compared to males.[23]

In a 2009 study published in the *Journal of Investigative Dermatology*, researchers in an effort to clarify the conflicting melanoma statistics analyzed the U.S. government's Surveillance Epidemiology and End Results (SEER) melanoma data covering the years 1992 though 2004. They determined that melanoma incidence rates doubled in all socioeconomic groups, all cell subtypes, and all thicknesses of the cancer upon diagnosis.[24] An analysis revealed that the increase in incidence of melanoma was a true increase in the actual number of cases, and not the result of more intensive screening due to increased public awareness of the malignant signs to look for in moles, and therefore having earlier diagnoses.[25]

From the 1960s to the present time there has been a steady rise in the incidence of melanoma in all parts of the world.[26] A 2009 study published in *Clinics in Dermatology* reveals the incidence rate for melanoma has been rising in White populations world-wide over the last four decades.[27] Statistics from the WHO estimate the annual incidence rate for melanoma in Norway and Sweden has more than tripled over the last 45 years.[28] Australia and New Zealand have the highest incidence rates at 40–60 per 100,000. Central Europe increased from 3–4 per 100,000 in the 1970s to 10–15 per 100,000 by 2000. These trends indicate that there will be a doubling of the incidence over the next 20 years.[29] In fact, the statistics are so overwhelming, researchers in a 2008 article published in the *European Academy of Dermatology and Venereology* stated: "it is probably safe to suggest that predominantly UVB absorbing sunscreens do not prevent melanoma development in humans."[30]

This result of increasing melanoma even with sunscreen use was identified in 1993 in an *Annals of Epidemiology* article by Dr. Garland and fellow researchers at University of California, San Diego. They concluded their study with the advice: "If melanoma and basal cell carcinoma are initiated or promoted by solar radiation other than UVB, as laboratory data suggest, then UVB sunscreens might not be effective in preventing these cancers, and sunscreen use might increase the risk of their occurrence." "Traditional means of limiting overexposure to the sun, such as wearing of hats and adequate clothing and avoidance of prolonged sunbathing, may be more prudent than reliance on chemical sunscreens."[31] Dermatology researchers at the Mayo Clinic even stated in a 1996 article in *Dermatologic Surgery* that:

". . . there is not a direct relationship between ultraviolet radiation and melanoma."[32] Yet, sunscreens have and still continue to be promoted as essential to protect us against melanoma.

Skin Cancers: Basal Cell and Squamous Cell Carcinomas

Sunscreens have been promoted for use due to the ability of solar rays to create changes to the DNA in the melanocytes that lead to melanoma and to the basal cells or squamous cells that lead to basal cell or squamous cell carcinomas, respectively. The most common form of skin cancer is basal cell carcinoma, which develops in the basal layer or deepest layer of the 5 layers of the skin's epidermis. This is the same layer that contains the melanin producing cells, the melanocytes. Squamous cell carcinoma is the second most common form of skin cancer, accounting for approximately 20% of the skin cancers. It arises from the squamous layer, which is the outermost layer of epidermis.[33] See Figure 1.

The U.S. National Institutes of Health does not keep track of the numbers of skin cancers that are caused by basal cell or squamous cell carcinomas the same as they do with melanomas. Therefore, only estimates regarding the prevalence of these skin cancers can be obtained by experts who run statistical analyses on pooled data bases. This method established the risk of having skin cancer in the U.S. in 1996 to be 1 in 5. They estimated that 97% of skin cancers would be nonmelanoma, or reaching approximately 1,000,000 cases of basal and squamous cell carcinomas. Out of this number, they predicted 38,300 melanoma cases.[34]

Studies based on individual practices help when looking at whether the incidence is rising or falling for these types of cancers. In a 2005 study published in *The Journal of the American Medical Association* (JAMA), doctors stated they found that the number of women under age 40 diagnosed with basal cell carcinoma had more than doubled in the previous 27 years (13.4/100,000 to 31.6/100,000), and the squamous cell carcinoma rate for women had also increased significantly.[35] A compilation of studies show that the incidences in basal cell and squamous cell carcinoma among predominantly White populations have increased continually since the 1980s. In a 1996 article in *Dermatologic Surgery*, the researchers stated the reason for their investigation was that: "The incidence of skin cancer is increasing at an alarming rate."[36]

Switzerland: Skin Cancer Rates Increasing

A 2009 study analyzing the incidence of skin cancers in Switzerland has identified that the rates for both squamous cell and basal cell skin cancers are increasing. Even though they have had a nationwide prevention campaign for the last 20 years, their rates are among the highest in Europe.[37]

Croatia: Skin Cancer Rates Increasing

In surveying Croatians, more than 70% of the population state they use sunscreens.[38] Even with all this use, the annual incidence of melanoma in Croatia has increased 300% over the last 40 years.[39] In fact, skin cancers are increasing so rapidly that a 2010 article written to promote the use of protective clothing to address this growing problem stated: "Skin cancer incidence in Croatia is steadily increasing in spite of public and governmental measurements. It is clear that it will soon become a major public health problem."[40]

The statistics do prove the increase in skin cancers of all types, and doctors are discussing amongst themselves this apparent contradiction of increasing sales of sunscreens paralleling an increasing incidence in skin cancers.[41]

What research is continuingly and universally revealing with the increase in skin cancers with the ubiquitous use of sunscreen chemical filters is an example of:

"The law of unintended consequences."

This law identifies that outcomes from a particular "thought to be good" action, which intervenes in a multipart system always generates unanticipated and often undesirable outcomes.

To date, it is clear that sunscreens are not providing the protection they have been promoted to do. To understand why this is happening, we need to look at:

1. The nature of the sun's rays (Chapter 3).
2. The affect of the chemicals used as sunscreen filters (Chapter 4).
3. Whether the sunscreens are capable of doing what they have been claimed to do (Chapter 5).

Chapter 3
The Sun's Rays

The identification of ultraviolet rays did not occur until 1801 by Johann Wilhelm Ritter. He identified the effects of light below the visible blue, calling it "infraviolet".[42] Since that time, much has been learned regarding the sun's rays. Today, they are divided by their wavelengths into ultraviolet (UV), visible, and infrared range (IR). The UV [meaning beyond the color violet of the visible spectrum] is subdivided into 3 groups, followed by the visible range of light, then the infrared range (IR) that is generally divided into 3 subdivisions the same as UV. The wavelengths of the solar radiation spectrum are shown in Table 2.[43]

Table 2.   **Solar Radiation Spectrum Frequencies**

Spectrum	Wavelengths	Also Known As
Ultraviolet range (UV)		
Ultraviolet C (UVC)	100 – 280 nm	
Ultraviolet B (UVB)	280 – 315 nm	
Ultraviolet A (UVA)	315 – 400 nm	
Visible range	400 – 700 nm	
Infrared range (IR)*		
Infrared A (IRA)	700 – 1,400 nm	(near or NIR)
Infrared B (IRB)	1,400 – 3,000 nm	(short wave IR)
Infrared C (IRC)	3,000 nm – 1 mm	(mid, long, far wave IR)

* Depending on the source, these ranges may vary.

nm = nanometer
mm = millimeter

Solar Radiation Penetrating the Earth's Atmosphere

When measured, the proportion of the sun's rays that come through the atmosphere as UV is only approximately 4%. The visible and the near infrared A (IRA) range of the sun's rays that penetrate through the earth's atmosphere make up 49% and 47%, respectively.

UV light is shorter in wavelength and higher in both frequency and energy than the visible spectrum. When it reaches the atmosphere, UV radiation reacts with oxygen creating the ozone layer above the earth. The UVC waves do not penetrate through the earth's atmosphere. Of the UV radiation that is able to pass through the ozone layer and continue coming through the atmosphere to the surface, 95-99% are in the UVA radiation range, while only 1-5% are the UVB part of the spectrum that the original SPF sunscreens were manufactured to filter out.[44] These percentages become important when examining the solar frequencies that sunscreen products have been designed to filter out. Most of the sunscreen formulations were made to filter the UVB, which are 1-5% of the 4% UV radiation reaching the surface of the earth. See table 3.

Table 3. **Radiation that Penetrates Earth's Atmosphere**

Solar Spectrum			
UV	4% →	UV Portion of Spectrum	
		UVC	0%
		UVB	1-5%
		UVA	95-99%
Visible	49%		
Near NIR (IRA)	47%		

What Happens When Our Skin Is Exposed to the Sun's Rays?

The UVB rays are what cause the reddening burn to the skin from prolonged exposure to the sun, which can damage and kill skin cells. This is the body's early warning system that is designed to alert you that the skin has had all the radiation it can maximally process without causing damaging changes. The reddening of the skin is actually due to increased blood flow into the damaged area as the body performs the process of healing itself by removing the dead cells. The pain from sunburns is caused by chemicals that are released from the damaged cells that activate the body's pain receptors.[45]

Chapter 4
Sunscreen Chemicals

How Do Sunscreens Work?

The original intent of manufacturers was to create products that prevented sunburns. Therefore, sunscreens were originally designed to protect only against the sun burning UVB rays. However, upon further investigation it is the UVA rays that are responsible for wrinkles and skin cancers. Formulations were then designed to shield from both UVB and UVA and became labeled "broad-spectrum" sunscreens. These are currently being promoted for the public to use because they cover more of the UV radiation range.

Recent research reveals that IR rays also lead to wrinkles and damage that can result in cancer, and as a result investigations into ways of preventing IR damage within the skin are only just beginning. More detail on IR is covered in Chapter 15.

Sunscreens, to date, are classified as either chemical (organic) absorbers or physical (inorganic) UV radiation blockers. Chemical filters are termed absorbers because they work by absorbing high-intensity UV rays. The original sunscreens were these absorbing chemicals that filtered just the UVB rays.[46] (Since none of the chemicals totally bock the sun's rays, they are termed *sun filters* rather than *sun blockers*.)

UVB Sunscreens

As shown in Figure 2, UVB rays only penetrate the epidermis layer of the skin. This penatration of the epidermis is what results in common the "sunburn".

Skin Penetration by UVB Solar Rays

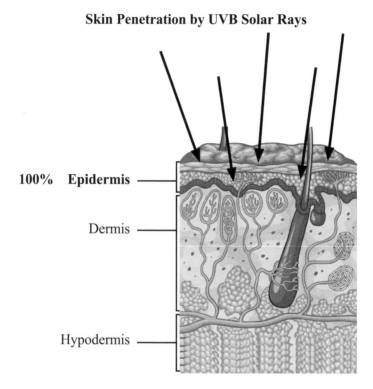

100%   **Epidermis** ——

Dermis ——

Hypodermis ——

Figure 2. Skin penetration of the epidermis by UVB radiation.

Many different types of chemicals are used in the manufacturing of sunscreens that protect against UV rays. Each chemical has its own range of solar radiation that it absorbs. None of them span the entire UV range, so manufacturers combine several chemicals together in order to provide protection from as much of the solar spectrum as possible.

The following are the chemical family groups that provide only UVB protection. They are listed so you can recognize their names when you are looking at the ingredients listed on products you intend to put on your skin.

UVB Only Filters

Camphors
  3-benzylidene camphor (3-BC)
  4-methylbenzylidene camphor (4-MBC) – also known by the names:
    Eusolex 6300
    Parsol 5000
    (Approved in Europe and Canada, not in U.S. or Japan).
Cinnamates
  Cinoxate
  Ethylhexyl methoxycinnamate (EHMC)
  Isopentyl-4-methoxycinnamate (IMC)
  Octinoxate – also known by the names:
    Eusolex 2292
    Octyl methoxycinnamate (OMC)
    Parsol MCX
PABAs
  Para-amino-benzoic acid (PABA)
  Esters of PABA:
    Ethyl-4-aminobenzoate (Et-PABA)
    Ethoxylated ethyl-4-aminobenzoate (Peg25-PABA)
    Glyceryl PABA
    Octyl dimethyl para amino benzoate (padimate O), (OD-PABA)
  (These modifications to PABA create less of an allergic reaction
  than with PABA itself, but this makes them less effective
  sunscreens than the original PABA.)
Parsol SLX – also known by the names:
  Dimethico-diethylbenzalmalonate
  Polysilicone-15
Salicylates
  Homosalate (HMS)
  Octyl salicylate, (octisalate), (OS) – also known by the names:
    Escalol 587
    Ethylhexyl salicylate

UVB Rays and SPF Labeling

To determine the SPF (sun protecting factor) that a particular sunscreen product is capable of providing, tests are performed in a laboratory to determine the amount of time people can spend in the sun and be protected from the reddening burn on the surface of the skin (the classic sunburn caused from excess exposure to the UVB rays). The SPF number indicates the amount of time a person can stay in the sun compared to no protection. For example, a SPF 30 denotes that a person can stay in the sun 30 times longer than normal without experiencing a burn.

The customary recommendation is for a sunscreen to have a SPF of at least 15, protecting the skin from 93% of UVB. The upgrade to a SPF 30 sunscreen only increases the protection to 97%, but doubles the amount of time people are told they can expect to be able to spend in the sun safely.

A major focus of the U.S. Food and Drug Administration's (FDA) investigations is to determine whether the product protects the body from the UV rays to the degree that the manufacturer claims it does. The new FDA guidelines issued June 2011 contained several changes. Rather than using the older terms of "water resistant" (40 minutes) and "very water resistant" (80 minutes), manufacturers are now required to state on the front of their labels how often they need to be reapplied after water contact. "Reapply after 40 [or 80] minutes of swimming or sweating; immediately after towel drying; at least every 2 hours."[47] For a more complete list of the guidelines see Appendix E.

Added into determining the effectiveness of a sunscreen is how long it will last under different conditions. Much of its effectiveness is lost from the impact of wind and the water that result from swimming, perspiring, or just humidity in the air. This is why sunscreen product labels recommend that they by reapplied at least every two hours. Also, there is a warning that using sunscreens along with an insect repellent can decrease its effectiveness. Further, just aging on the shelf can decrease its effectiveness, and it is recommended that bottles over 2 years old be thrown away.[48]

Why UVA Sunscreens

The reason that there has been such an urging to cover every part of the skin with a sunscreen before going into the sun is due to the fact that ultraviolet wavelengths have the ability to penetrate the skin and cause damage at the molecular level. The SPF rating only applies to a sunscreen's ability to filter UVB rays; it does not apply to its ability to screen out UVA rays also.

UVB radiation is fully absorbed by the outermost top layers of the epidermis as was shown in Figure 2, while for those with fair Caucasian skin, 50% of UVA radiation penetrates through the layers of the epidermis and deep into the dermis layer underneath. See Figure 3.

Skin Penetration by UVA Solar Rays

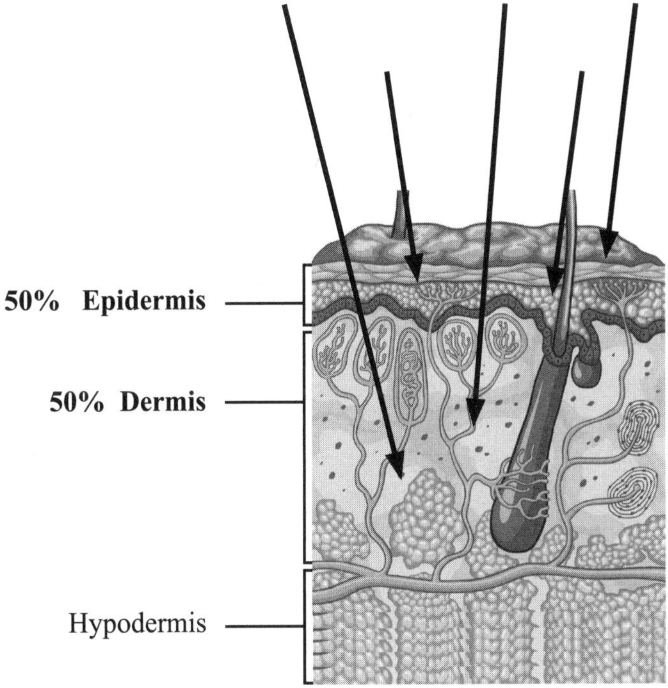

50% **Epidermis**

50% **Dermis**

Hypodermis

Figure 3.   Skin penetration of the epidermis and dermis by UVA radiation.

The penetration of UVA waves into the dermis becomes critical when more than 95% of the sun's ultraviolet light coming through the atmosphere reaches us in the UVA frequency range. It is even more important as these rays penetrate much deeper, and when they enter the skin to the dermal layer they are then free to generate what are termed reactive oxygen species (ROS). The ROS are unstable molecules containing oxygen that function as free radicals, which are capable of causing cellular damage.[49]

The chemicals utilized for sunscreens cannot dissipate the energy as efficiently as the body's own built-in defense, melanin, which is the brown pigment that is made by the melanocytes in the basal layer of the skin. The use of sunscreens stops the body's natural process of creating more melanin to naturally protect the cells. The use of UVB only sunscreens, allowing people to stay in the sun longer, does not stop the UVA rays from penetrating into the lower layers of the skin where they create a greater increase in the amount of free radicals and ROS than would have occurred without the use of sunscreen. Experiments show sunscreens protect for the first 20 minutes, but after 60 minutes the three sunscreen chemicals octocrylene (OC), the cinnamate OMC, and benzophenone BP3 actually generate more ROS in the skin compared to using no sunscreen.[50]

ROS: Cause Cancer

Reactive oxygen species are highly chemically-reactive molecules because the oxygen molecules they contain have unpaired electrons. They are the natural by-product of oxygen metabolism in the body's tissues, and normal levels of ROS created by routine body processes can be handled by normal levels of antioxidants, which the body utilizes to neutralize the ROS. Environmental stress like UV radiation absorbed into the skin increases ROS levels significantly. Increased antioxidants are then necessary to protect the skin from what is termed photo-oxidative stress, which causes damage to cell membranes,

DNA, chromosomes, lipids, and proteins. This leads to inflammation and suppression of the immune system and results in increased risk of melanoma, as well as basal and squamous cell carcinomas.[51]

Studies show that blocking both UVB as well as strong protection from UVA (SPF 25, plus a UVA protection factor of 14) is necessary to prevent the increase in ROS.[52] Recognition of this made researchers realize sunscreens that protect from reddening of the skin without including comparable protection from the deeper penetrating UVA rays has made the incidence of skin cancer greater than ever, as both UVB and UVA filters had been necessary to have any affect on decreasing cancer.[53] Studies have proven that UVA radiation has the ability to lead to squamous skin cell carcinoma as well as melanoma. Researchers have determined this by the fact that squamous cancer cells contain UVA signature mutations; and have also found that UV radiation frequencies produce melanoma in fish.[54]

ROS: Cause Photoaging

Rather than protecting the skin to keep it young looking, not filtering UVA radiation leads to greater photoaging. Increases in ROS destroy the collagen and elastin, which are protective chemicals that keep skin firm. Collagen and elastin are our friends in our skin that provide the framework and elasticity that keep the skin supple and young looking. Without collagen providing strength, the skin becomes thinner. Elastin supplies a matrix that holds individual skin cells in place. Both of these are essential, and without the collagen and elastin, the skin starts to wrinkle and sag. When collagen and elastin are lost due to damage from light, it is called photoaging.[55]

The urging of sunscreen use has led to a false sense of security. People believing they are protected have been staying in the sun much longer than they normally would since sunscreens by-pass the skin's built-in warning system — turning red when the body is getting more radiation than its antioxidant level can handle. The increased amount of time in the sun generating excessive ROS has led to much more significant damage in the skin at the molecular level than before the use of sunscreens.[56]

Physical Filters: Reflect and Scatter UVB and UVA Rays

On recognizing that UVA rays cause more damage to skin cells than UVB rays, sunscreen manufacturers looked for chemicals that would filter out the UVA in addition to the UVB rays. Fewer chemicals have the ability to filter UVA rays so they had to turn to the physical or what they term the inorganic metals of titanium dioxide (TiO_2) and zinc oxide (ZnO). [Titanium oxide in its natural state has 2 oxygen molecules so there is a 2 on the O for oxygen in its scientific notation of TiO_2, whereas zinc oxide only has one oxygen molecule making its scientific notation ZnO.]

Both of these metals reflect, scatter, and absorb UVB rays, as well as absorb UVA. The ZnO absorbs the full UVA spectrum, while TiO_2 absorbs only the shorter UVA radiation frequencies. Since they are metals, they also have less potential for allergic skin reactions as experienced with some of the UVB filtering chemicals.[57]

Eliminating the White Cream Appearance

However, a major drawback of these physical filters is that both TiO_2 and ZnO leave a thick white residue on the skin. To avoid this undesirable effect, manufacturers drastically reduced the size of TiO_2 and ZnO down to very tiny "nano" sized particles. This reduction in size makes them more transparent to the eye, and the cream easier to apply to the skin. The nanoparticles are defined as those less than 100 nanometers (nm) and range in size from 10–50 nm compared to the nonmicronized "bulk" form that is much larger at 200–500 nm. Although nano-sizing them makes their use much more acceptable by the public, the decrease in size also decreases the amount of the

UV spectrum they screen out, which reduces their effectiveness as sunscreens.

In 1999, the FDA allowed nano-sized particles to be used in sunscreens. There are no requirements in the U.S. that sunscreens, cosmetics, or any products that contain them to be labeled whether they contain nano or bulk sized particles. This technology has been adopted around the world. By 2006, nano-sizing took off so well in Australia that 70% of TiO_2 and 30% of ZnO sunscreens were formulated with nanoparticles rather than the bulk size of the metals.[58]

Chemicals that Provide Only UVA Protection

To date, there are few chemicals that filter UVA rays. As various names for each are utilized by different manufacturers, their alternate names are listed so you can identify them when checking the lists of product ingredients. UVA filtering chemicals are:

Avobenzone – also known by the names:
  BMDBM
  Butyl methoxydibenzoylmethane
  Escalol 517
  Eusolex 9020
  Parsol 1789
Mexoryl SX – also known by the names:
  Ecamsule
  Terephthalylidene dicamphor sulfonic acid
Uvinul A Plus – also known by the name:
  Diethylamino hydroxybenzoyl hexyl benzoate

Manufacturers have not been able to find or create a chemical that protects against the full spectrum of the sun's rays. Many versions and combinations of UV filtering chemicals have been created to address the difficulties that each chemical has on its own. Among the problems are: a narrow range of the UV spectrum that is screened out; a tendency to elicit allergic reactions; water soluble and wash off easily; become inactivated by exposure to sunlight; while others induce unwanted reactions when mixed with other chemicals. They each have their own solubility and whether they combine well with other chemicals depends on if they are water or lipid (fat) soluble. Therefore, the goals manufacturers have been attempting to deliver in a sunscreen are:

Covers the entire UV spectrum.
Does not wash off.
Does not cause allergic reactions.
Does not degrade and become inactive in sunlight.
Does not interact with other chemicals that:
Reduce their effectiveness.
Create new harmful chemical complexes.

Since no one chemical provides all of these qualities, more and more chemicals and combinations of chemicals have been created in the attempts to reach these goals. As a result, there has been much research to develop one chemical that accomplishes the attributes listed above that are needed in a single sunscreen. Many chemicals have been developed in their search, as none of them have the ability to supply all the aspects necessary.

Chemicals that Provide UVB Plus Some UVA Filtering
There are a few chemicals that in addition to filtering some of the UVB radiation also provide some UVA protection. The chemicals are listed below by their chemical family groups.

UVB plus UVA Filtering
Benzophenones
Benzophenone-1 (BP1)
Benzophenone-2 (BP2)
4-hydroxy benzophenone (4HB)

4,4'-dihydroxybenzophenone (4DHB)
Benzophenone-3 (BP3)– also known by the names:
   Oxybenzone
   2-benzoyl-5-methoxyphenol
   2-hydroxy-4-methoxybenzophenone (HMB)
   2-hydroxy-4-methoxyphenyl-phenylmethanone
   Advastab 45
   Anuvex
   Chimassorb 90
   Cyasorb UV 9
   Escalol 567
   Eusolex 4360
   MOB
   Spectra-Sorb UV-9
   Sunscreen UV 15
   Syntase 62
   UF 3
   Uvinul 9
   Uvinul M-40
   Uvistat 24
Benzophenone-4 (BP4) – also known by the names:
   Sulisobenzone
   Escalol 577
Benzophenone-8 (BP8) – also known by the name:
   Dioxybenzone
Mexoryl XL – also known by the names:
   Dometrizole trisiloxane
   Terephthalylidene dicamphor sulfonic acid
Octocrylene (OC)
Tinosorb S – also known by the names:
   Bemotrizinol
   Escalol S

UVB Plus Miniscule UVA
PBSA – also known by the names:
Ensulizole
Eusolex 232
Parsol HS
Phenylbenzimidazole 5-sulfonic acid

Combinations that Provide Broader UV Coverage
Tinosorb M – also known by the names:
Bisoctrizole
MBBT: methylene-bis-benzotriazolyl tetramethylbutylphenol:
A hybrid of an organic chemical plus physical blocker of nanoparticles between 100–200 nm in size. It is highly stable, and utilized to stabilize other UVB blockers that are not stable in sunlight.[59] (One 2001 study showed it did not have estrogenic effects in either laboratory analyses or in rats.)[60]
Anthelios SX (U.S.) combines:
Mexoryl SX (ecamsule) for short UVA rays
Parsol 1789 (avobenzone) for long UVA rays
Octocrylene (OC) for UVB rays

As of June 2011, the FDA now states that only sunscreens that pass the FDA broad spectrum test procedure that measures UVA relative to UVB protection and have a SPF value between 15 and 50 may label their product as: "Broad Spectrum SPF 15 (50)".

Considering it has taken decades and hundreds of studies to finally identify that most of the sunscreen chemicals and physical blockers approved over the last 30 years cause harm, it would be wise to wait until more studies have been completed before utilizing these new chemicals. In an effort to avoid recreating the harm to humans and to the environment that has been allowed to occur with the sunscreens marketed to date, extensive testing needs to be completed before allowing more mass marketing and distribution of these new chemicals.

Chapter 5
U.S. FDA – Approvals and Regulations

World-wide there is a difference in how sunscreen chemicals are treated. In Europe, they are treated as cosmetics, whereas in the United States (U.S.) they are regarded as drugs so they fall under the regulation of the Food and Drug Administration (FDA). As a result, there are 27 chemicals allowed to be utilized and sold in sunscreens and cosmetics in Europe compared to 16 chemicals approved in the U.S.

The FDA began regulating sunscreens for safety and effectiveness in 1978. The following time-line highlights the regulations as adopted by the FDA.

1978 – Proposed regulations of the UVB filtering sunscreen chemicals, with recommended standards for safety and effectiveness. Created and established guidelines for UVB SPF testing and labeling.

1988 – Approved the chemical avobenzone, a UVA-only filter, as a sunscreen product. Avobenzone was patented in 1973 and approved for use by the European Union (EU) in 1978. Before avobenzone, the FDA approved filters only stopped UVB rays and had no or only incidental UVA protection.[61]

1990s – National Laboratories Created:
By the 1990s, FDA awareness of the increased incidence of skin cancers led to the establishment of new laboratory facilities devoted to phototoxicology and photocarcinogenesis. Three centers for the National Toxicology Program (NTP) were created: the NTP Center

for Phototoxicology; the Interagency Center for the Evaluation of Alternative Toxicological Methods; and the Center for the Evaluation of Risks to Human Reproduction.[62]

1997 – Allowed sunscreen makers to market that their products contain avobenzone for UVA protection.

2006 – Approved ecamsule, a UVA and UVB filter as a new drug application (NDA).

NDA approval means that federal regulations permit the ingredients to be used in combinations for over-the-counter (OTC) sunscreen and cosmetic products without premarket approval as long as each active ingredient contributes an SPF of at least 2, and is within the concentration limits that are allowed.[63]

2006 – Missed a deadline established by Congress to approve proposed standardized guidelines for sunscreens.

2007 – Asked for public comments on their finalized proposed rules for testing and labeling UVA filters, and their recommendations for suntanning safety. Their proposed guide would implement new standardized testing and labeling practices to clear up the confusion over UVA ratings. It also was looking to determine if products did what their advertising claimed such as: lasting all day; being waterproof; or protecting as a broad-spectrum filter by screening out both UVA and UVB rays.[64]

2009 – The National Toxicology Program (NTP) reported they were investigating titanium dioxide (topically and intradermally applied) and a mutation in the tumor suppressor gene called p53, which was appearing to be involved in skin cancer development.[65]

2010 – Ecamsule Pediatric Safety NDA Approval

FDA Memorandum (January 6, 2010):

> U.S. New Drug Application 2006/2008 for adults, children greater than 6 months old with partial waivers granted for children less than 6 months of age, allowing ecamsule to be marketed as OTC final monograph ingredients (21 CFR 352).

> Anthelios 40 sunscreen cream (Helioblock SX) contains 4 active ingredients with 4 combinations of varying concentrations of: ecamsule; avobenzone; octocrylene; and TiO_2 nanoparticles.

The FDA approves this combination use of ecamsule without full data as to its safety, as it recognizes the other 3 ingredients as safe and have been available.

All OTC sunscreens, whether regulated by the monograph or the NDA process described above, are currently labeled for use for children down to 6 months of age.[66]

2010 – The FDA stated they would announce their new policy guidelines by October, 2010. The FDA states the reason for the delay is due to the great quantity of research that needs to be evaluated, as well as the substantial amount of feedback they received regarding the 2007 proposed guidelines.[67]

2011 – June 14: New guidelines for product labeling were announced in regards to water resistant claims and UV spectrum claims, as well as strength of filtering the radiation. See Appendix E for details.[68]

There have been no requirements by the FDA for sunscreens to undergo animal toxicity testing to determine whether the absorption of the chemicals could lead to either general or reproductive toxicity. The chemicals that have been approved to date were approved before the studies on possible gestational impact were performed.[69]

Why UVA Ratings Have Taken So Long

A major problem with determining how well a filter protects the skin from UVA rays is due to the fact that it is very difficult to measure the protectiveness it may offer from UVA wavelengths. With UVB rays causing sunburn, the endpoint is easy to measure. Since UVA rays do not create a burn or cause immediate visible damage, it is difficult to find an endpoint that would provide a measurable scale to determine the amount of UVA radiation that a sunscreen chemical would allow through the skin. So far there is no consistent grading system that is used. One test that has been used is a change in pigmentation, rather than a change in reddening as with UVB. This measurement is called the "persistent pigment darkening" (PPD) method, which identifies the amount of UVA radiation that creates a persistent darkening or tanning of the skin. However, there are too many variables that can change the results to make this a consistent and reliable grading scale.[70]

As to whether a label for UVA protection should be added to sunscreen packaging, researchers, themselves, state they question the ability of the public to understand and grasp its complex structure and meaning well enough for it to be worthwhile. One study ended with the words: "Finally, there is evidence that the consumer has yet to come to grips with the concept of SPF. Thus, it may not be useful to add another rather specialized protection index (a UVA rating scale)."[71] The U.K. and Ireland have developed a UVA rating system called the Boots Star Rating system that started out as a 4 star and was revised to a 5 star system, because they eliminated 1 and 2 stars after determining they would be too weak to offer enough protection.

Under this system a product with a 5 star rating would provide the highest UVA/UVB protection. The June 2011 U.S. FDA guidelines announced that the star system rating would not be required, just the SPF combined rating that would include UVA and UVB.[72]

With these systems in place, the increased use of sunscreens provides a false sense of security resulting in people staying in the sun much longer than they normally would. The problem is that it is much longer than the body can naturally absorb and process the sun's rays without causing either short or long-term damage. The difficulty this creates is highlighted in the conclusion of a 2010 article published in *Archives of Dermatological Research* that stated:

". . . excessive and chronic exposure to UV radiation can overwhelm the cutaneous (skin) antioxidant capacity, leading to oxidative stress and oxidative damage which may result in skin disorders, immunosuppression, premature aging of the skin and development of melanoma and non-melanoma skin cancers."[73]

In other words, these researchers have identified that the body cannot process the excess exposure to the sun's rays that results from sunscreens allowing people to stay in the sun longer than normal without a breakdown in its many systems, which could include the development of skin cancers.

Part 2 – Chemical Sunscreens

Chapter 6
Testing Chemicals for Toxicity and Safety

New sunscreen chemicals are brought to market without complete testing of their potential for toxicity toward the environment, their action within the body, or whether they can be passed through to the fetus and thereby affect the next generation. One reason studies are lacking in regards to our bodies is that the gold standard of scientific testing, the double-blind study, cannot be performed on humans with chemicals that are of an unknown nature that could potentially be toxic and cause harm.

Earth's Ecosystem and Body's Biochemistry: Complexity We Cannot Begin to Comprehend

In testing whether sunscreen chemicals are safe for use on the planet there are many difficulties that have to be taken into account in determining whether outcomes and conclusions from the studies can be relied upon. The body's biochemistry is so complex it is impossible to design studies that identify, much less have the ability to accurately measure, all the effects one particular chemical may have when it enters the body of humans, fish, corals, or the earth's entire ecosystem.

In the 21st century, each organism is exposed to such an accumulative plethora of chemicals and environmental effects, it is very difficult to isolate the impact of just one chemical in a laboratory setting. Current evidence is revealing that the chemicals do not act alone. There is now such a complex sea of environmental chemicals, when they interact together they become much more toxic than if there was just one. Yet, we continue to test for the affect of just one chemical and its reaction as if it were acting alone, which does not take into account the many chemicals that are within each living organism.

Chemical Family Groups

Today, topical or systemic toxicity that could result from long-term use remains unresearched for many skin care ingredients, including sunscreen chemicals. In reality, there are so many sunscreen chemicals on the market, there is no ability, nor enough money, to test each one of them to the fullest extent that would necessarily include years of accumulated use, as well as gestational studies on all of them. This drawback can be overcome by looking at the broader picture. All chemicals belong to families based on their having the same basic structures, which results in their having the same characteristic behaviors and actions at the biochemical level. Testing how one chemical from a particular family group acts at the cellular level can be applied to other chemicals from that particular family group, as they would be expected to have the ability to cause the same effects.

This book breaks out and discusses the sunscreen chemicals by the name of the chemical family to which they belong. In looking into their potential effect on humans, as well as the environment, if one chemical from a particular chemical family causes a particular effect, then it is far better to be cautious and assume that the very slightly different structure of a chemical from the same family group would have the potential for causing the same effect. When one from a group is identified as toxic, until it is proven otherwise, all from that group need to be avoided until there is sufficient proof they will not harm life on the planet.

Drawbacks of Chemical UV Sunscreen Filters
Allergic Reactions

The earliest sunscreen chemical PABA created problems because of the many people who developed skin allergies with its use. This was very common and much research was conducted to modify the PABA molecule to reduce its propensity to trigger the allergic reactions. The sunscreen chemicals known to cause higher percentages of allergic skin reactions are:

PABA
Avobenzone
Oxybenzone (BP3)

Researchers are identifying an increasing number of allergic responses to oxybenzone, also commonly known as BP3. There have now been several cases where it has caused an anaphylactic response. This is a great risk as anaphylactic reactions can result in death without immediate treatment. If there are allergic type symptoms, this should be considered a possibility for someone who has applied sunscreen, or even touched clothing that has been on skin to which sunscreen has been applied. People have reported that putting on the same bathing suit months later led to another allergic reaction.[74]

Photo Instability
UV Radiation Can Cause Sunscreen Chemicals to Breakdown
On exposure to sunlight, not all chemicals retain the ability to protect the skin by absorbing or reflecting the UV radiation. Some sunscreen chemicals are classified as "photo stable". That is they stay intact and continue to provide filtering of the solar spectrum even after sun exposure. While there are others that breakdown when exposed to sunlight and are termed "photo unstable". When they breakdown, they no longer offer protection from the sun's UV radiation. All chemicals are investigated for the amount of stability they exhibit when exposed to sunlight and are chosen based on their ability to remain stable. If they are not stable in sunlight, yet filter a part UV radiation that others do not, they are mixed with chemicals that are stable to create a product that is capable of retaining its effectiveness when exposed to sunlight.

Photo Unstable Sunscreen Chemicals
Benzophenone: Oxybenzone (BP3)
Cinnamates:
Octinoxate
Octyl methoxycinnamate (OMC)
Parsol MCX
Avobenzone
Approved for use in the U.S. in 1988, avobenzone is so unstable in sunlight that research proves that by itself, it does not protect skin cells from undergoing harmful stress and death.[75] Manufacturers have to mix it with other chemicals for it to have any ability to filter the UV rays.[76] However, the sunscreen chemicals that it necessarily needs to be mixed with can be toxic, and additionally there can be unexpected chemical reactions between them that can cause harmful effects. Combining it with TiO_2 or ZnO nanoparticles actually accelerates its photo degradation.[77]

Photo Stable Sunscreen Chemicals
Mexoryl SX – also known by the name:
Ecamsule
[Even though it appears to be relatively non-toxic and has rarely caused skin irritation, research has not included gestational studies or studies on its body-wide effects.][78]
Mexoryl XL
Salicylates
Weak UV screens, but due to being so photo stable they are added to unstable UV filters to stabilize them.
Tinosorb M bisoctrizole
Tinosorb S bemotrizinol
Uvinul A Plus – also known by the name:
Diethylamino hydroxybenzoyl hexyl benzoate

Researchers state that it is a fine balancing act to create a formula that will cover the full UV spectrum in an emulsion that will spread evenly on the skin and also be photo stable, and at the same time not penetrate into the outer layer of the skin. The difficulty is detailed in the following opening to a study published in 2010:

"The preparation of commercial products able to protect the skin against damage from solar radiation requires safe and photo-stable UV-absorbing molecules with high extinction coefficients, prepared with solvents of the appropriate polarities and polarizabilities in formulas which allow the uniform spreading of the UV-absorbing substances. The products should also maintain the ingredients on the top of the skin and provide efficient scavenging activities against singlet oxygen and other directly or indirectly generated reactive oxygen species (ROS). Because of the high doses of UV used to test high SPF, simple and reproducible methods are needed to estimate the protection afforded by the product before risking the induction of severe burns to the volunteers, as can occur when the value of the product's SPF is smaller than the expected one."[79]

These researchers clearly feel that any chemical placed on the skin should be designed to not be absorbed. In the same study, they also state that education of the public in the proper use of sunscreens (e.g., to be applied every 2 hours, etc.) is essential to guarantee that it does provide the protection they are claiming.

Chapter 7
Endocrine Disrupting Chemicals (EDCs)

There have been so many new chemicals brought to market, especially in the last half of the 20th century, that disrupt normal endocrine (hormone) function they have been given their own label: Endocrine Disrupting Chemicals or EDCs. Many EDCs have the ability to disrupt normal hormone functioning because they are so similar in structure they can take the place of the organism's own hormones, which can create an excessive response, or prevent the body's natural hormones from carrying out their essential functions. To determine the effect these chemicals have on the skin as well as in the body, it is necessary to look at how they act at the biochemical level.

When they act like an estrogen (female hormone) or an androgen (male hormone), they can have an impact on sexual characteristics and reproductive functions. Chemicals can not only mimic estrogens and androgens, they can also act against them. When they disrupt or inhibit the action of these hormones, the chemical is described as anti-estrogenic, or anti-androgenic. There have been many lab experiments, as well as animal studies published over the years that demonstrate that the UV filters used as sunscreens and in cosmetics are capable of exhibiting all four of these types of actions: estrogenic; androgenic; anti-estrogenic; and anti-androgenic activity.

Sunscreen Chemicals are EDCs
Benzophenones

In 1983, an expert panel reviewing the literature available at the time published a "Final Report on the Safety Assessment of Benzophenones-1, 3, 4, 5, 9, and 11" that stated:

"On the basis of the available animal data and clinical human experience presented in this report, the Panel concludes that Benzophenones -1, -3, -4, -5, -9, and -11 are safe for topical application to humans in the present practices of use and concentration in cosmetics."

This was the conclusion even though the body of the article had the following statements:

" . . . another study showed benzophenone-3 (BP3) at 0.5% was toxic."

"No information was available on any of the Benzophenones with respect to teratogenesis (toxicity causing defects and malformations to the developing fetus) and carcinogenesis (causing cancer)."[80]

Benzophenones have been widely used in many products based on reports like this that concluded they are safe for humans to use. But were these conclusions premature? Based on this 1983 final report on their safety, there were no studies identifying the possibility of their leading to either birth defects or cancer.

Let us look at the evidence that is available today. What do the studies that have been conducted since these sunscreens were declared safe for use reveal?

Benzophenones belong to a class of chemicals called phenols. Studies over the years have proven that phenols are well absorbed from the gastrointestinal tract and through the skin of both animals and humans.[81]

Bisphenol A (BPA) and benzophenone-3 chemical structures are very similar as illustrated in Figure 4.

Chemical Structure of Bisphenol A (BPA) and Benzophenone-3 (BP3)

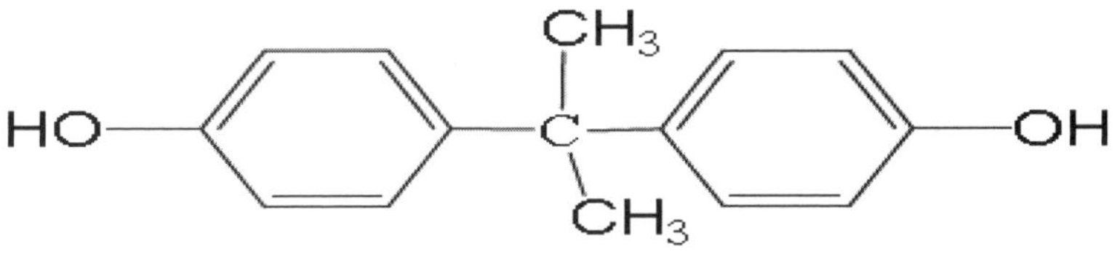

Bisphenol A (BPA)

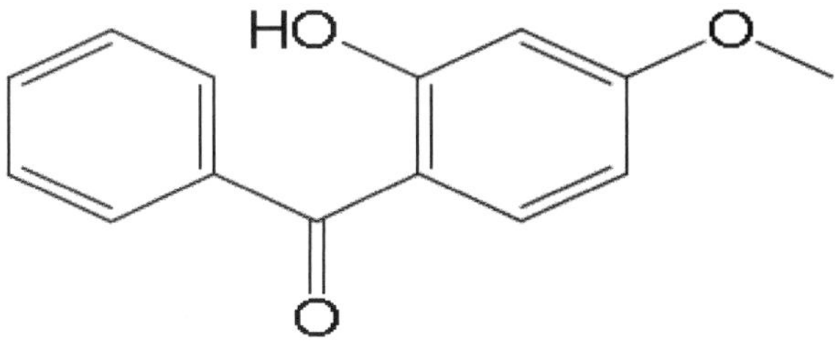

Benzophenone-3 (BP3)

Figure 4. Chemical structure of bisphenol A (BPA) and benzophenone-3 (BP3).

Since they are of the same chemical group, they can be expected to demonstrate similar characteristics and actions at the cellular level. The phenol bisphenol-A (BPA) is a well known estrogenic EDC that is commonly found in plastics, which due to its hormonal estrogenicity the U.S. National Institutes of Health National Toxicology Program (NTP) has concluded there is evidence to have "some concern" over effects on the brain, behavior, and prostate gland in fetuses, infants, and children at current levels of exposure.

One group of researchers investigating sunscreens found that all 18 of the sunscreen chemicals they tested exhibited hormonal activity.[82] The sunscreen chemicals tested were:

Benzophenones
    BP1
    BP2
    BP3
    BP4
    4DHB
    4HB
Camphors
    3-BC
    4-MBC
Cinnamates
    IMC
Octocrylene (OC)
OMC (Parsol MCX) PABAs
    PABA
    Et-PABA
    OD-PABA (padimate O)
    PEG25-PABA
Salicylates
    BS
    HMS
    OS
    PS

Sunscreen Chemicals: Impact on Mammals

Benzophenone-3 (BP3)
Mice: General and Reproductive Toxicity

Research started in 1988 and completed in 1991 tested the potential influence of low, medium, and high doses of BP3 for hormone activity in mice. The mice were then evaluated for general and reproductive toxicity. Their results published in 1997 showed that the mice exhibited the following changes:

Table 4.   **Mice: General Toxicity**

	Change	Dosage
First Generation Adverse Effects:		
Body metabolism*		
Male weight reduced by	8%	high
Female weight reduced by	13–18%	med / high
* Even though food intake increased at all doses.		
Second Generation Adverse Affects (only high dose measured):		
Body metabolism		
Male weight reduced by	14%	
Female weight reduced by	11%	
Liver		
Male liver weight increased	50%	
Female liver weight increased	30%	
Kidney		
Female kidney weight increased	10%	

Table 5   **Mice: Reproductive Toxicity**

	Change	Dosage
First Generation Adverse Effects:		
Females - Pregnant		
Decease in number of living		
pups per litter	22–23%	med / high
Days to litter increased*	7–11%	high
Pup weight reduced	7–10%	med / high
Females - Nursing		
Unexpected deaths**		all doses
Pups died because		
mothers died	30–33%	
Remaining pups		
Lower body weights	20-40%	med / high
Second Generation Adverse Effects (only high dose measured):		
Males		
Testicles weight reduced	6%	
Prostate weight increased	30%	

* Some stopped having litters altogether.
** With no signs of illness.

The researchers summarized their findings stating they found BP3:

Reduced pup weight.
Reduced the number of pups per litter.
Increased mortality of nursing females at doses that reduced body
    weight.
Increased liver and kidney weights.

These results demonstrate that this common sunscreen chemical affects the entire body, including the liver and kidneys, as well as disrupts normal reproductive development and subsequent generations.[83]

Benzophenone-2 (BP2)

A 2004 study on rats determined that BP2 is a hormone disrupter in multiple organ systems throughout the body. Researchers compared the effects of the strongest human ovarian estrogen (E2: estradiol), with BP2 for their influence on the uterus, vagina, pituitary, liver, and HDL and LDL metabolism. After only 5 days of treatment with BP2, the rats demonstrated hormonal changes similar to those created by the E2 human estrogen.[84]

Rats: General and Reproductive Toxicity
Estrogenic changes were observed in:
Body weight.
Food intake.
Increased uterine weight.
Increased growth factor protein (Igf1) in the vagina and in the liver.
Reduced luteinizing hormone (LH) synthesis in the pituitary (LH influences menstrual cycle and androgen production).
Reduced cholesterol, HDL, and LDL.
Thyroid hormones:
T4 and T3 levels significantly reduced.
(The researchers theorized the decreased thyroid hormones could be the result of BP2 inhibiting thyroid peroxidase (TPO), the enzyme that is essential for the formation of the thyroid hormones.)

Benzophenones, Camphors, Cinnamates
Rats: Reproductive Toxicity

A study published in 2001 looked at the affect of 6 chemical sunscreens given orally or applied to the skin of immature rats on uterine weight measurements. The chemicals tested were the:

Benzophenone: BP3
Camphor: 4-MBC
Cinnamate: octyl-methoxycinnamate (OMC)
Homosalate: HMS
PABA: OD-PABA

Using the well known estrogenic hormone birth control ethinylestradiol (EE) and estradiol E2 as controls, 3 out of the 6 chemical sunscreen UV filters tested were found to increase uterine weight in immature rats. This demonstrates that these chemicals exerted estrogenic activity in the tissues of the rats.

Oral feeding for 4 days.
    Uterine weight increased by:
        4-MBC
        OMC
        BP3 (weakly)

Skin application of 4-MBC also increased uterine weight

Based on these results the researchers stated concern that: "Our findings indicate that UV screens should be tested for endocrine activity, in view of possible long-term effects in humans and wildlife."[85]

In 2004, these same researchers published findings of their further investigations into estrogenicity of sunscreen chemicals.[86] Again, looking at the affect on immature rats in the laboratory, this time using the known estrogenic hormone birth control ethinylestradiol (EE) as a control, 6 out of 9 chemical sunscreen UV filters tested were found to increase uterine weight, which also demonstrates that they exert estrogenic activity in tissues. The chemicals that increased uterine weight were:

BP1
BP2
BP3
4-MBC
3-BC
OMC

Anti-androgenic Hormone Effects

When a chemical acts like an anti-androgen, blocking androgenic or male hormone activity, the action would have a similar effect as having estrogenic activity. In testing for anti-androgenic activity, this study identified 2 anti-androgenic chemicals.

Anti-androgenic activity was demonstrated by:
BP3
HMS
No anti-androgenic activity was shown by:
BP4, 3-BC, 4-MBC, OD-PABA, OMC, avobenzone
(BP1 and BP2 were not tested in this study)

Showing estrogenicity stronger than the human estrogen estradiol (E2) by displacing E2 from the human estrogen receptor were:

3-BC
4-MBC

Thyroid Toxicity
Increased thyroid weight by:
4-MBC

Camphors
Rats: Reproductive and Developmental Toxicity
Also investigating the effects of the camphors 4-MBC and 3-BC given orally to pregnant rats they found:

Pregnant females:
   3-BC
      Decreased weight
Male and female offspring changes:
   4-MBC and 3-BC
      Delayed male puberty
      Increased reproductive organ weights of adult male and female
      Female sexual behavior decreased
   4-MBC
      Altered development in:
         Hypothalamo-pituitary-gonadal system
         Estrogen-regulated gene expression in reproductive organs [The toxicity was seen at tissue concentration levels of 4-MBC that approach the range of UV filters that have been found in fish in Swiss lakes.][86]

After further investigations of the same sunscreen chemicals in 2008, these researchers determined that both the reproductive organs and the central nervous system demonstrate they are sensitive targets that develop toxic developmental effects from the hormonally activating sunscreen chemicals. They concluded: "These data indicate that pre- and postnatal exposure to 4-MBC and 3-BC can interfere with sexual development at brain and reproductive organ levels."

They also determined that differing combinations of chemicals appear to affect the type of influence they exert.

The researchers stated their results, combined with evidence that there is a bioaccumulation (build up) in wildlife and humans, highlight a need for comprehensive analyses of the toxic potential of sunscreen chemicals, especially in regards to reproduction and development in offspring.[87]

In 2007, other researchers found similar results when they fed 4-MBC to rats during pregnancy, lactation, and for 12 weeks into adulthood.

Oral feeding of 4-MBC to pregnant and lactating rats:
Male offspring demonstrated
 Delay in puberty
 Decreased prostate weight
 Changed reactions to estrogen

They concluded their data indicate that pre- and postnatal exposure of 4-MBC in rats interferes with male sexual development.[88]

Further confirmation of 4-MBC interference in reproductive development was published in a 2008 *Environmental Health Perspectives* study that found giving 4-MBC and 3-BC to pregnant rats results in a significant increase in tissue volume in the prostate and accessory sex glands in the developing fetal rat.[89]

Cinnamates
Octyl-methoxycinnamate (OMC)
 A 2010 *Toxicology and Applied Pharmacology* article examined pregnant rats that were given 3 dosage levels of OMC. The females were tested for hormone levels and juvenile offspring were tested for both hormone levels and sexual organ development. The crucial thyroid hormone, T4, at gestation day 15 in the pregnant mothers

measured at 26.5 nM in the control, a value that dropped to 7.1 nM at the low dose, 0.6 nM at the medium, and 1.0 nM at the highest dose of OMC. At day 15 post delivery in the nursing mothers, the control was 16.0 nM, low dose OMC was 4.8 nM, medium was 0.6 nM, and high dose was 0.0 nM T4. This means that there is not enough thyroid hormone for the proper neurodevelopment of the fetus or juvenile offspring during its crucial early brain development, which could result in lifelong alterations in neuropathways. These as well as other outcomes this study identified are listed below.

Rats: Thyroid, Developmental, and Reproductive Toxicity
T4 Significantly Decreased at All Doses in:
  Pregnant Females at
    15 days gestation (a critical time of fetal physical and neural development.)
  Nursing Mothers at
    15 days post delivery
  Offspring at 16 days
    Male

Developmental Effect in:
Male and Female Offspring at 16 Days
  Body weight
    Significantly decreased – high dose
  Thyroid gland weight
    Significantly increased – med & high doses
  Liver weight
    Significantly increased – med & high doses

Reproductive Sex Hormones Effect in:
Male and Female Offspring at 16 Days
    Testosterone
        Significantly reduced – dose dependently (the higher the dose,
        the greater the reduction)
Male and Female Offspring at 28 Days
    Progesterone
        Significantly decreased – all doses
    Estradiol levels
        Significantly decreased – low & med doses

Reproductive Organ Changes in:
Male Offspring at 16 Days
    Testicle weight
        Significantly decreased – med & high doses
    Testicle development
        Significantly delayed – high dose
    Sperm count
        Significantly lowered – all doses
    Prostate weight
        Significantly decreased – high dose
    Prostate
        Microscopic changes in development – dose dependently

Male Offspring Adult at 8 Months
    Sperm count
        Significantly lowered – all doses
    Prostate weight
        Significantly reduced – high dose
    Prostate atrophy – med & high doses

These researchers concluded that OMC is not only estrogenic, it is also anti-thyroid. They expressed there is cause for worry over the fact that the OMC resulted in lowered sperm counts at all dosage levels since lowered sperm counts have been identified in humans over the last few decades. Finding that reproductive and neurological development of rat offspring are adversely affected led the researchers to conclude that their results: ". . . maybe a cause of concern, as humans are systematically exposed to this compound though usage of sunscreens and other cosmetics."[90]

Chapter 8
The Aquatic Environment

EDC Sunscreen Chemicals Impact on Fresh Water

When sunscreens are applied to the skin, they wash off into the water, as well as wash off of the clothes people wear, and subsequently enter the aquatic environment. Since these chemicals are shown to exert hormonal influences in laboratory assays as well as in animal studies on rodents, it is necessary to look at what affects the sunscreen chemicals may have on the fish that live in the water we swim in after slathering our bodies with sunscreens. Additionally, since we excrete these chemicals out in our urine and feces, we need to determine whether wastewater treatment plants have the ability to sufficiently remove them.

There is reason for concern about chemicals accumulating in our waterways. Korean researchers suspecting contamination of the water supply that comes from surface waters sampled water from upstream and downstream of the Han River and from effluent-dominated creeks along the river. They tested for 31 compounds and frequently detected the sunscreen chemical benzophenone, the drugs naproxen, carbamazepine, caffeine, and the insect repellent DEET.[91]

Impact on Fish
EDC Sunscreen Chemicals Accumulate in Fish

The mass use of sunscreens has led to their being detected in water sources everywhere, and research is uncovering that the sunscreen chemicals that are now in our lakes and rivers can accumulate in aquatic organisms. Table 6 shows the concentrations of the different sunscreen chemicals found in the lakes, rivers, and oceans of various countries throughout the world. The table also identifies that the chemicals are found in the muscles of the fish that swim in these waterways. The sunscreen chemicals detected were:

4-MBC (4-methylbenzylidene camphor)
BP3 (benzophenone-3)
EHMC (2-ethyl-hexyl-4-trimethoxycinnamate)
OC (octocrylene)
BM-DBM (avobenzone or 4-tert-butyl-4-methoxydibenzoylmethane)
Et-PABA (ethyl-4-aminobenzoate)
4HB (4-hydroxybenzophenone)
HMS (homosalate)
DHB (2,4-di-hydroxybenzophenone)
OTC (Uvinul T 150 or octyl triazone)

Table 6.
Concentrations of UV Filters in the Environment and Biota (fish)

Environmental Sample	UV Filter	Max. Concentration [ng/l, mg/kg dw]	Location / Ref
Lake water	4MBC	80	Switzerland[92]
	BP3	125	
	EHMC	19	
	OC	27	
	BM-DBM	24	
	BP3	85	Slovenia[93]
	EHMC	92	
	Et-PABA	34	
	OC	31	
	4HB	85	Korea[94]
River water	HMS	345	Slovenia[93]
	BP3	114	
	EHMC	88	
	OC	34	
	DHB	47	Korea[94]
Seawater (beach)	4MBC	488	Norway[95]
	BP3	269	
	EHMC	238	
	OC	4461	

Table 6 cont.
Concentrations of UV Filters in the Environment and Biota (fish)

Environmental Sample	UV Filter	Max. Concentration [ng/l, mg/kg dw]		Location / Ref
Raw drinking water	EHMC	5610		California[96]
Raw wastewater	4MBC	6500		Switzerland[97]
	BP3	7800		
	EHMC	19000		
	OC	12000		
	BP3	6240		California[96]
	EHMC	400		
Treated wastewater	4MBC	2700		Switzerland[97]
	BP3	700		
	EHMC	100		
	OC	270		
Swimming pool water	4MBC	330		Slovenia93
	BP3	400		
Fish (lakes)	4MBC	3.80	mg/kg (lw)	Germany[98]
	HMS	3.10	mg/kg (lw)	
	EHMC	0.31	mg/kg (lw)	
	BP3	0.30	mg/kg (lw)	
	4MBC	0.17	mg/kg (lw)	Switzerland[97]
	BP3	0.12	mg/kg (lw)	
	EHMC	0.07	mg/kg (lw)	
	OC	0.02	mg/kg (lw)	
Fish (rivers)	4MBC	0.42	mg/kg (lw)a	Switzerland[99]
	OC	0.63	mg/kg (lw)a	
Sewage sludge	4MBC	1.78	mg/kg (dm)a	Switzerland[100]
	EHMC	0.11	mg/kg (dm)a	
	OC	4.84	mg/kg (dm)a	
	OTC	5.51	mg/kg (dm)a	

a mean concentrations; dw, dry weight; lw, lipids weight; dm, dry matter.

Source: Fent K, Kunz PY, Gomez E. UV filters in the aquatic environment induce hormonal effects and affect fertility and reproduction in fish. Endocrine disruptors: natural waters and fishes. *Chimia*. 2008. 62(5):368-375. Reprinted with permission.

Residues of the sunscreen chemical groups of camphors, cinnamates, benzophenones, and salicylates, in the form of 4-MBC, OMC, BP3, and HMS are found in muscle tissue of perch and roach (carp), as well as in whitefish from a lake in Switzerland.[101] The Swiss adopted a nationwide preventive campaign of protecting the skin and utilizing sunscreens. These high concentrations of sunscreen chemicals found in their waterways confirm the effectiveness of their campaign. Yet, they still have steadily increasing skin cancer incidence rates as discussed in Chapter 2.

Reproductive Toxicity: Intersex Fish
Estrogenic Sunscreen Chemicals and Preservatives

Multiple studies by many researchers are showing reproductive changes in various species of fish. The estrogenic chemicals disrupt their hormonal development, and ultimately interfere with their ability to reproduce. When researchers investigate environmental chemicals to determine whether a chemical acts like an estrogen, they utilize a marker protein that is a precursor protein of egg yolk called vitellogenin or VTG. Normally VTG is found only in the blood or circulatory fluids of females, but upon exposure to estrogenic chemicals, males are found to have the same elevated levels as females. These EDC exposed fish are neither completely male nor completely female, so scientists have labeled them "intersex fish" to describe their abnormal reproductive developmental outcomes.

Benzophenones
BP2: Estrogenic

Swiss researchers published a study in 2007 revealing that the benzophenone, BP2, impacts minnow's reproductive capabilities. BP2 accumulated in the fish and exerted estrogenic effects on secondary sex characteristics, gonad development, and reproduction. They found that males produced the egg yolk protein VTG in a dose dependent manner (the amount of VTG produced increased as the dose of BP2 increased). Reproduction was negatively affected, as both sperm in the males and egg development in the females was significantly inhibited. Reproduction was impacted to the point that some even stopped spawning completely.[102]

BP3: Estrogenic

Exposing rainbow trout and Japanese medaka rice fish to BP3 induced the production of VTG and resulted in significant impairment of their reproduction. The researchers stated there is a propensity for rapid accumulation of BP3, with the environment reaching the concentrations that impact egg development in the fish.[103]

Benzophenones and Camphors
BP1, BP2, 3-BC: Estrogenic

Multiple research studies clearly demonstrate BP1, BP2, and 3-BC are estrogenic. Researchers in Switzerland exposing fathead minnows to these chemicals for 14 days found all 3 sunscreen chemicals exerted estrogenic effects, as demonstrated by the induction of VTG being produced by male fish.[104]

Camphors, Cinnamates, and Preservatives
4-MBC, OMC, Propylparaben: Estrogenic

Japanese researchers exposed Japanese medaka rice fish to the camphor 4-MBC, the cinnamate (OMC), and propylparaben (PP). The PP is commonly used in sunscreen formulas as a preservative and antimicrobial agent. They found all 3 chemicals show estrogenic activity as there was VTG development in the male fish.[105]

PAPA: Estrogenic

Even the PABA chemicals that were utilized in the first sunscreens, which have been around a long time, have demonstrated a propensity for estrogenicity also. After 14 days of exposure to the PABA derivative, Et-PABA, VTG production was induced in fresh water juvenile fathead minnows.[106] Figure 5 shows VTG production is created not only by Et-PABA, but also by 3-BC, BP1, and BP2.

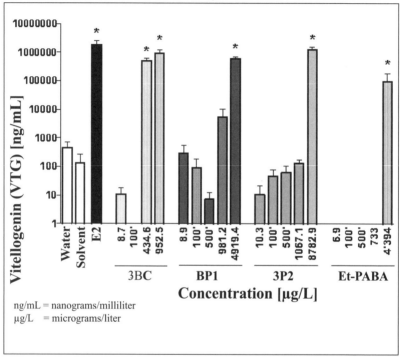

Figure 5. Estrogenic activity of UV filters after exposure of juvenile fathead minnows for 14 days. As a biomarker for estrogenic activity, vitellogenin (VTG) in fish was determined. Benzophenone-1 (BP1), benzophenone-2 (BP2), 3-benzylidene camphor (3-BC) showed estrogenic activity.

Source: Fent K, Kunz PY, Gomez E. UV filters in the aquatic environment induce hormonal effects and affect fertility and reproduction in fish. Endocrine disruptors: natural waters and fishes. *Chimia.* 2008. 62(5):368-375. Reprinted with permission.

The graph illustrates that the camphor 3-BC, the benzophenones BP1 and BP2, as well as the PABA Et-PABA all have the capacity to produce as strong an estrogenic response as the strongest human estrogen, estradiol or E2. They are all capable of generating approximately 100,000 ng/mL VTG.

Sunscreen Chemicals Exert Multiple Hormonal Influences

UV filters are being shown to have multiple hormonal activities. In addition to the estrogenic (female) effects researchers have seen, they are uncovering they also exert androgenic (male) effects, as well as block or oppose the effects of estrogens or androgens, exhibiting anti-estrogenic and anti-androgenic effects respectively.

Hormones work throughout the tissues of the body by attaching to a receptor in the cell that is specific for each hormone. When a chemical attaches to a receptor, it exerts influences that are for its specific hormonal activity. When a chemical attaches to an estrogen receptor, it has the capability to function like an estrogen. When it attaches to an androgen (testosterone) receptor, it could function like an androgen. If it blocks the activity of a natural estrogen or androgen, then it acts as an anti-estrogen or anti-androgen, respectively.

The hormonal influences that sunscreens display are shown in Table 7. The more pluses that are shown under each type of hormonal influence, the greater the hormonal activity the sunscreen exerts in the tissues that are influenced by hormones, and the ### signs demonstrate the greatest activity. This table shows that not only do these chemicals act like female hormones (estrogenic activity), which would impact male fish, their influence can have even greater impact on male fish because they also exert an affect that opposes male hormone influence (anti-androgenic activity). Female fish are also impacted as the chemicals can exert influence against female hormones, which is shown as anti-estrogenic activity and androgenic activity as demonstrated in Table 7.

Table 7.   **Sunscreen Reactivities with Estrogen (female)
And Androgen (male) Cell Receptors***

Compound	Estrogenic Activity	Anti-estrogenic Activity	Androgenic Activity	Anti-androgenic Activity
4-Methylbenzylidene camphor (4MBC)	---	+++	---	###
3-Benzylidene camphor (3BC)	+	+++	---	###
Benzophenone-1 (BP1)	+++	---	---	###
Benzophenone-2 (BP2)	+++	---	+++	###
4-Hydroxy benzophenone (4HB)	###	---	---	###
4,4'-Dihydroxybenzophenone (4DHB)	###	---	---	###
Benzophenone-3 (BP3)	+	+++	---	###
Benzophenone-4 (BP4)	+	+++	---	+++
Isopentyl-4-methoxycinnamate (IMC)	---	+++	++	###
Ethyl hexyl methoxycinnamate (EHMC)	---	+++	++	###
Octocrylene (OC)	---	+++	+	###
Benzyl salicylate (BS)	+	###	---	+++
Phenyl salicylate (PS)	++	+++	---	###
Homosalate (HMS)	---	+++	+++	###
Octyl salicylate (OS)	---	+++	++	###
Para amino-benzoic acid (PABA)	---	+++	---	---
Ethyl-4 amino benzoate (Et-PABA)	###	---	---	++
Octyl dimethyl para amino benzoate (OD-PABA)	---	+++	---	###
Ethoxylated ethyl 4-amino benzoate (Peg25-PABA)	---	+	---	---

+++ = Maximal dose-response curves with ≥ 80% efficacy.
++ = Submaximal dose-response curves with ≥ 30% efficacy.
+ = Submaximal dose-response curves with < 30% efficacy.
= Most potent hormonal activity found for each compound.
--- = Not detected.

Sources: Fent K, Kunz PY, Gomez E. UV filters in the aquatic environment
induce hormonal effects and affect fertility and reproduction in
fish. Endocrine disruptors: natural waters and fishes. *Chimia*.
2008. 62(5):368-375. Reprinted with permission.

* Kunz PY. Fent K. Multiple hormonal activities of UV filters and
comparison of in vivo and in vitro estrogenic activity of ethyl-4-
aminobenzoate in fish. *Aquat Toxicol*. 2006. 79:305.

Researchers in France found that the benzophenones BP1, BP2, and BP3 all show anti-androgenic activity. In addition, one of the forms that benzophenone turns into in the body, the metabolite THB, shows even greater anti-androgenic activity than its parent benzophenone.[107] Other researchers testing the effects of anti-androgens in the Japanese medaka fish stated the results of their study indicate that fish become "intersex" when exposed to anti-androgens, with the potential of altered testicular development, as well as altered sperm and egg development.[108]

Other researchers found the benzophenone metabolite, THB, in the highest concentration in the liver, followed by the kidneys, spleen, and testicles. These results indicate that there is a body-wide distribution of the sunscreen chemicals once they are absorbed.[109]

Benzophenones and Salicylates
BP1, BP2, BP4, PS, and BS: Anti-androgenic
Hormonal disruption is displayed by the benzophenones BP1, BP2, BP4, and 2 different salicylates, phenyl salicylate (PS) and benzyl salicylate (BS). All of these sunscreen chemicals demonstrate more anti-androgenic (disruption of male testosterone) activity than that of flutamide, the anti-androgen given to prostate cancer patients to stop the influence of testosterone in the effort to slow prostate cancer growth.[110]

Combining Sunscreens to Improve Entire UV Spectrum Coverage
Since most UV sunscreens now utilize many chemicals in their formulas to cover the entire UV spectrum, researchers are expressing growing concerns over the possibility that, even at low concentrations of each one individually, the accumulation of many different sunscreen chemicals may act together causing even greater alterations in fish reproduction.[111] A 2007 study published in *Environmental Science & Technology* looking into whether the UV filtering chemicals could act together in an accumulative manner revealed that they do have the capacity to act together to affect reproductive performance, even

though the level of each component, by itself, is so low it is below the threshold of measurable effects.[112]

In 2010, researchers looking into this effect examined 4-MBC, EHMC, BP3 and BP4 on *Daphnia magna* (water flea). They found the low level of each one by itself did not pose a problem, but that mixed together the chemicals demonstrated an additive effect. They concluded that the mixture of these occurring in surface waters may pose a toxic risk in the ecology for sensitive aquatic organisms, and they recommended that UV filters undergo further analysis of possible cumulative toxic effects, since the studies on sunscreen chemicals to date have not ruled out their risk to the environment.[113]

This cumulative toxic effect that arises due to the blending of the many chemicals illustrates how imperative it is to stop these chemicals from entering the waterways of the world to begin with, as many are accumulating in our lakes and rivers as shown previously in Table 6.

Do Wastewater Treatment Plants Remove the Sunscreen Chemicals?

A 2006 study examining fish from seven Swiss rivers that receive water from waste treatment plants found the sunscreen chemicals 4-MBC and octocrylene (OC) in the muscle tissue of brown trout in higher concentrations than those found in fish from lakes (whitefish and roach fish). The researchers believe this identifies that wastewater treatment plants that dump filtered water from human wastewater into rivers are major sources for the sunscreen chemicals that are found in the aquatic environment.[114]

A 2010 study from Switzerland found the same concentrations of BP4, BP3, 4-MBC, and the cinnamate (EHMC) above and below waste treatment plants, showing that wastewater treatment plants do not remove these chemicals that are washed off while swimming or bathing, or excreted in urine. They also found the evidence that there may be a food-chain accumulation, as EHMC was found in 48 invertebrate and fish samples from six different rivers, as well as in 5 cormorants (aquatic birds) from the same area.[115]

Chapter 9
EDC Sunscreen Chemicals – Impact on Humans

The U.S. Government Occupational Safety and Health Administration (OSHA) has required Material Safety Data Sheets (MSDS) on all hazardous materials since 1986. An excerpt from one that has been written for benzophenones is presented in Table 8 below.[116]

Table 8.   **OSHA: MSDS – Benzophenone**
(Diphenylmethanone; phenyl ketone; Diphenyl ketone; Benzoylbenzene)

The toxicological properties of this substance have not been fully investigated.
Label Hazard Warning: WARNING! HARMFUL IF SWALLOWED OR INHALED. CAUSES IRRITATION TO SKIN, EYES AND RESPIRATORY TRACT. AFFECTS CENTRAL NERVOUS SYSTEM.
Use with adequate ventilation. Avoid contact with eyes, skin, and clothing. Avoid ingestion and inhalation.
Inhalation: Causes respiratory tract irritation.
Skin: Causes skin irritation. Animal feeding studies have resulted in liver and bone marrow damage.
Ingestion: Ingestion of large amounts may cause gastrointestinal irritation.

Table 8 cont.   **OSHA: MSDS – Benzophenone**
(Diphenylmethanone; phenyl ketone; Diphenyl ketone; Benzoylbenzene)

Eyes:	Wear appropriate protective eyeglasses or chemical safety goggles as described by OSHA's eye and face protection regulations in 29 CFR 1910.133 or European Standard EN166.
Skin:	Wear appropriate gloves to prevent skin exposure.
Clothing:	Wear appropriate protective clothing to prevent skin exposure.
Environmental Toxicity:	This material may be toxic to aquatic life.

These warnings illustrate that benzophenones can be toxic, not only to our health, but also to the earth's ecosystem. We need to be conscious consumers by protecting our bodies and those of our children from the possible chemical toxicity of these chemicals that are being added to the products we use daily.

Skin Penetration

A study published in 2000 in the *American Journal of Clinical Dermatology* stated that the extent to which sunscreens are absorbed into deeper tissues, and therefore into the blood and circulated systemically over time, is currently unknown. Much depends on the formulation of the vehicle that the sunscreen is suspended in, as each base and combination of chemicals have significantly differing effects on the absorption into the skin.[117] Studies on the potential for penetration of the sunscreen chemicals through the skin have found that many are absorbed and distributed throughout the body.

Oxybenzone or Benzophenone 3 (BP3)

BP3 has been used for more than 30 years by millions of consumers on a daily basis. In addition to sunscreen lotions, it has been incorporated as a UV filter into lipsticks, lip balms, facial moisturizers, hair sprays, dyes, and shampoos. It is also used in the manufacture of antihistamines, hypnotics, insecticides, and because it protects scents and colors from UV light damage, it is added to heavy perfumes, and soaps.

Since it is utilized in products that are applied to the lips, and therefore very likely to be swallowed, researchers tested whether it is absorbed by the GI tract by feeding BP3 to rats. In 1993, studies on oral administration of BP3 to rats showed that it is rapidly absorbed, being detected in the blood 5 minutes after exposure. In 6 hours after administration, both BP3 and the products it turns into (metabolites) are in most tissues of the body, with the highest concentration in the liver.[118]

In another study published a year later, the same researchers in applying BP3 on the skin of male rats, found BP3 in their blood 5 minutes after administration, with peak concentrations found 2½ hours later. They also found the liver to have the highest concentration, followed by the kidneys, spleen, and testicles.[119] Further investigations allowed these researchers to identify that BP3 given orally to male rats was excreted in the urine, as well as through the feces.[120]

It not only absorbs rapidly, the body does not release it all, and as a result it builds up in the body. In 2006, when Swedish researchers had human volunteers apply BP3 body-wide for 5 days, they found that it accumulates in the body as only an average of 3.7% of the amount applied was excreted in the urine when they were followed and tested 5 days after their last application.[121]

Widespread exposure to BP3 and the inability of the body to excrete it all is evidenced in a study testing the blood of the U.S. general population during the years 2003 and 2004 that showed BP3 was found in 97% of the samples. Women and Whites had the highest concentrations, showing over 1,000 µg/g (micrograms per gram) creatinine. The pervasiveness of BP3 throughout the population was further demonstrated by testing the blood of adult volunteers who claimed they had no exposure to BP3. Even though they stated they had not used sunscreens, over 90% of them were also found to have BP3 in their blood.[122]

Skin penetration and absorption of the benzophenone BP3, the cinnamate OMC, and the camphor 4-MBC was confirmed in male and female volunteers. All three chemicals were found in the volunteer's blood and urine. This study also confirmed that the body does not get rid of the chemicals; rather they accumulate in the tissues as concentrations were greater at 96 hours after exposure to the chemicals compared to the levels attained at only 24 hours after exposure.[123]

The cinnamate (also known by the names octinoxate, octyl methoxycinnamate (OMC), and Parsol MCX) is also systemically absorbed through the skin. Concern over skin penetration has led to researchers looking into finding new routes and formulations that would limit the amount of their absorption.[124]

In investigating whether there is skin penetration from spray applications, testing the aerosol of the newer sunscreen filter Tinosorb (MBBT) and the cinnamate EMC showed that these chemicals do absorb through the skin.[125] Spray application is also accompanied by the possibility of inhaling the chemicals through the lungs, since it is difficult not to breathe the vapors of the aerosolized chemicals as they are being applied to the skin. Once in the lungs, they have direct and easy access to the bloodstream.

Since manufacturers are combining many of the sunscreen chemicals in order to cover as much of the solar spectrum as possible, it is important to look at whether there is a possibility of greater skin penetration. Each chemical by itself may not penetrate the skin easily, but researchers looking into the possibility of whether combinations of chemicals have greater penetration do find they cross much more readily into the skin when several are grouped together.[126]

Children's Skin Absorbs More than Adult Skin

A very important point to consider, since parents are urged to slather their children with sunscreen, is that children and babies have a greater ratio of skin surface area to body weight. Additionally, their skin is more porous and permeable than adults, who have thicker and tougher skin. So a smaller amount of chemical put on children's skin leads to their absorbing and attaining much higher blood levels when compared to that of adults.[127] What may appear as a small amount for an adult, results in a much greater dose for a child with less body mass.

Sunscreen Chemicals: Found in Household Dust

The sunscreen chemicals are now so ubiquitous that they are even found in household dust vacuumed from private homes. In a 2009 article published in *Journal of Chromatography*, researchers testing household dust found octocrylene (OCR), the cinnamates EHMC and IAMC, the salicylate EHS, and the camphor 4-MBC. This means that we are not only absorbing them through the skin, we are also breathing them in through our lungs from the day-to-day dust found in our homes and workplaces.[128]

Since 97% of Americans now have BP3 in their blood, what is the potential impact on our bodies?

Sunscreen Chemicals: Found in Breast Milk

Since phenols are readily absorbed following inhalation, ingestion, or through skin contact, they become widely distributed throughout the body, including into human breast milk, resulting in their transfer to the babies who are breast fed. In a 2006 study of 20 breast milk samples that were tested for phenol compounds, researchers identified 3 different chemicals in over 60% of the samples. The sunscreen chemical BP3 was in 60%, bisphenol A (BPA), which is incorporated into many plastics and plastic bottles including baby bottles, nipples, and pacifiers was in 90%, and ortho-phenylphenol (OPP), a germicide and fungicide used on citrus fruits and vegetables, was in 85% of the positive samples.[129]

In a study published in 2010, researchers performed an analysis of the combined results of studies on breast milk from the years 2004, 2005, and 2006. By 2006, sunscreen chemicals were present in 85% of the human milk samples. The highest concentrations were from BP3, followed by OCT, HMS, EHMC and 4-MBC. Increase in use of sunscreens is seen in the repeated sampling across time. In 2004, OCT was found in 54% of the samples, but only 2 years later (2006) it was in 100% of the positive samples. In 2004, the sunscreen chemical 4-MBC was only in 7.7% of the samples, but its prevalence increased to 35% of the samples by 2006. HMS was non-existent in 2004 and 2005, and then appeared in 29% of the samples by 2006. These results show that the sunscreen chemicals are very absorbable and may accumulate over time, and that our babies are drinking in and absorbing these chemicals on an ever increasing basis.[130]

The U.S. has a National Toxicology Program (NTP) that is a division of the Department of Human Health Services within the National Institutes of Environmental Health Sciences (NIEHS), which are all under the National Institutes of Health (NIH). In 2007, a panel of 12 independent scientists was commissioned by the NTP Center for the Evaluation of Risks to Human Reproduction (CERHR) to assess scientific studies on the potential reproductive and developmental hazards of bisphenol A (BPA). ". . . the Panel concluded that the overall findings suggest that bisphenol A may be associated with neural changes in the brain and behavioral alterations related to sexual dimorphism in rodents. For this reason, the Panel expressed 'some' concern for these effects even though it is not clear the reported effects constitute an adverse toxicological response." Their conclusion was that it was of "negligible" concern for adverse reproductive effects. For highly exposed subgroups, such as occupationally exposed populations, the level of concern was elevated to "minimal". For infants and children they stated ". . . some concern for neural and behavioral effects, and minimal concern for accelerated puberty."[131] These conclusions of the NTP give cause for concern as a 2010 study just 2 years later shows that BPA could cause developmental harm, creating not only metabolic changes in the body, but also behavioral disorders.[132]

Indeed, studies examining sunscreens and their effectiveness or potential harmful consequences demonstrate conflicting results that researchers, themselves, state are difficult to explain.[133] The major reasons for these inconsistencies are due to the fact that the human body and the interactions of the ecosystems are so complex it is difficult to design studies that can control all the individual and environmental variables in order to discern definitive answers.

Phenols Cross the Placenta

There is proof that the phenol BPA crosses the placenta, even at low environmental levels. Since benzophenones are phenols, it stands to reason they cross the placenta also, which means they could impact fetal development.[134]

Can We Learn from the Synthetic
Estrogen Diethylstilbestrol (DES) Debacle?

We have already tragically seen that it can take decades for the adverse effects from endocrine disruptors to show up as happened with the synthetic estrogen diethylstilbestrol (DES), which was initially introduced in 1938 to prevent miscarriages.[135] Between 1938–1971, 5 to 10 million women were prescribed DES during pregnancy, exposing millions of developing fetuses to this hormonally active chemical. It was not until 15 years later that research, published in 1953, showed that DES did not prevent miscarriages or premature births. Yet even with the proof that it was not beneficial, it was continued to be prescribed to millions of women. It was not until over 30 years later (1971) that the Food and Drug Administration (FDA) banned its use during pregnancy as result of a study published that year identifying DES could cause a rare form of vaginal cancer. It was continued to be used in Europe until 1978.[136]

DES was used to fatten livestock. When workers experienced the symptoms of sterility and breast growth, as well as the DES being detected in the livers of chickens, it was outlawed in 1959 for use chickens and lambs.[137]

However, it was still allowed to be used in cattle until 1979. This ubiquitous use led to over 80% of the cattle being exposed to the chemical and to it becoming part of our food supply, as well as to it being released into the environment through the cattle's waste.[138]

DES did not provide the protection that it was claimed to do. Even though it did not prevent miscarriages, it was still sold for decades, impacting millions with the potential adverse affects on the developing fetus. Allowing over 30 years of use led to profound consequences to humans and the environment. Not only did it not prevent miscarriages, it resulted in great reproductive harm. DES prompted late spontaneous abortions, and resulted in a higher risk of unsuccessful pregnancies, as well as ectopic (tubal) pregnancies. Children born to mother's taking DES had higher risk of cancers, reproductive organ abnormalities, higher rates of unsuccessful pregnancies, and lower sperm counts. There were also psychological disorders identified with greater rates of depression, learning disabilities, and anorexia. A study published in 2011 identified that the effect can continue transgenerationally finding that grandsons of women given DES during pregnancy have a higher incidence of the male reproductive organ disorder of hypospadias (male urethra opening on underside of penis).[139]

History has proven that these outcomes were predictive from the animal studies that were performed. Developing tissues, whether animal or human, are similarly impacted by hormone disruptors.

The same has happened with sunscreens. We have many species of fish showing the hormonal reproductive organ disruption caused by sunscreen chemicals. Sunscreens have not protected from skin cancers, yet are still being sold to millions around the world, even though they are demonstrating that they, too, can have adverse affects on developing embryos. Can we learn from history and take sunscreens off the market and out of the environment before the full impact of the harm they have the potential of causing to human fetal development comes to full identification years down the road?

The problem with waiting until the full potential of harm to show itself, rather than take heed to the mounting pile of evidence that sunscreens are estrogenic disrupting chemicals, was expressed in a study published in 2009 by one set of researchers who stated their concern:

"While research surrounding this topic is not conclusive, particularly in humans, there is certainly sufficient evidence to warrant concern about potential long term effects in both wildlife and humans. Obtaining absolute proof of endocrine disruption by BPA, phthalates, and other compounds with weak hormonal activity in humans is likely impossible because it would obviously be unethical to conduct a double-blind study where one group is exposed to a suspected toxicant. Research in animals, however, is robust and indicates that disruption of sex specific behavior, neuroendocrine circuitry and physiology is possible and, in some cases, transgenerational (being passed onto children and grandchildren)."

"The ability of these compounds to permanently affect the epigenome (expression of genes) could be potentially catastrophic to the welfare of future generations and requires further attention by both toxicologists and endocrinologists."[140]

Impact on the Human Fetus

Are sunscreens impacting unborn babies? Since it is unethical to run the usual scientifically accepted double-blind studies on humans, we have to look at other parameters to judge whether our unborn babies are being hormonally impacted. Researchers have had to find creative ways to measure the impact that these hormone disrupting chemicals might have on human fetal development. One parameter they have measured is newborn birth weights. When measuring maternal blood levels of BP3, researchers found higher BP3 concentrations are associated with increased birth weight in boys, but lower birth weight among girls.[141] This shows BP3 could be affecting fetal growth.

If we are seeing changes in male/female differentiation from the phenol compounds in the reproductive development in fish, what about the potential for changes in human fetal reproductive development, since phenols can cross the placenta and move into the developing baby?

Reproductive Development and Behavior Affected
Sexually Dimorphic Brain Development

During the development of the fetus, the sex hormones of testosterone and estrogens create profound organizational effects on the developing brain. As the testicles develop, they secrete the testosterone that is essential for the masculinization process responsible for the development of adult male sexual behavior, as well as exerts influence on defeminizing or decreasing the area responsible for adult female sexual behavior. This hormonal influence results in what scientists call an adult sexually dimorphic brain physiology that leads to male patterns of adult sexual behavior. In other words, during fetal development, when these hormone sensitive areas of the brain are bathed in estrogenic hormones, such as the sunscreen chemicals, rather than testosterone, the brain does not develop the normal male and female differentiation that results in patterning of gender specific adult sexual behavior.[142]

In a 2007 review of the scientific literature, Italian researchers wrote: "It has become increasingly clear that environmental chemicals have the capability of impacting endocrine (hormone) function. Moreover, these endocrine disrupting chemicals (EDCs) have long term consequences on adult reproductive function, especially if exposure occurs during embryonic development thereby affecting sexual differentiation."[143]

There are many environmental endocrine disrupting chemicals today and they all may be contributing to the changes that are being seen. The studies show that the affects are additive and even small amounts of each chemical, when added together create toxic changes.

Sunscreens Disrupt Testosterone

A 2010 study published in *Biochemical Pharmacology* reveals the need to research chemicals at the reproductive level. Swiss researchers looking for answers to the steadily increasing prevalence of male reproductive disorders and testicular cancer studied endocrine disrupting chemicals (EDCs) and their targets of action. They examined the effects of the sunscreen chemicals benzophenone BP1 and the camphors 3-BC and 4-MBC on an enzyme that is essential for the last step of testosterone synthesis in the testicles, and is required for male sexual development.

They found the camphors 3-BC and 4-MBC, as well as the benzophenone BP1 inhibit an enzyme that is necessary for testosterone production. This results in the inability of androstenedione [testosterone precursor] to be converted into testosterone.

In addition, even when there is sufficient amount of testosterone present, BP1 blocks the ability for it to act at the cellular level by preventing it from landing on the testosterone receptor of the cell. The result is the needed action of this male hormone cannot take place.

The researchers felt their findings on these disruptions to the proper functioning of the essential hormone, testosterone, by BP1, 3-BC and 4-MBC demonstrated that further investigation is required and should be considered as part of any safety assessment of these chemicals.[144]

EDCs Impact on Mammal Sexual Development

Animal studies show us that the potential for sunscreen chemicals to affect sexual differentiation of the fetus is quite probable. As stated earlier, researchers in 2004 identified the sunscreen camphor 4-MBC exerted an estrogenic influence on rat embryos that affected development of the endocrine hypothalamo-pituitary-gonadal (HPA) system of both male and female offspring. It changed estrogen regulated gene expression in their reproductive organs, as well as in the regions of the brain that exhibit sexual differentiation and are critical for enabling the adult to function either as a male or a female. The researchers warned that the pattern of developmental effect differs when several chemicals are combined, and the chemicals should be carefully evaluated in the context of multiple chemical mixtures.[145]

Mice

Experiments with mice show that the phenol BPA, an environmental estrogen, affects both female and male mouse brains during early development. Estrogen mimickers act differently and circumvent the normal route of protection during brain development. This means that estrogen mimickers can enter regions of the developing female brain that are normally protected from excessive estrogen exposure, potentially altering the expected developmental plan. The researchers state there is reason to be concerned about the daily exposure that is occurring while studies are still underway to fully understand the depth and breadth of the impact these estrogen-like chemicals have on fetal male and female brain differentiation.[146]

There have not been similar studies performed for BP3. However, since both BPA and BP3 are from the same chemical family, the phenols, and they both are environmental estrogens that can cross the placenta. From a biochemical point of view, it is reasonable to assume that BP3 has a similar impact on the developing brain.

In 2005, researchers stated: "The problem of endocrine disrupting chemicals (EDCs), i.e., chemicals that have the capacity to interfere with the endocrine system, has gained increasing attention as it has become clear that these environmental contaminants may be active in humans, as well as in wildlife and domestic animal species."

In looking at toxicological effects of EDCs, evidence is appearing that the estrogenic compounds may exert deleterious effects, even some time after exposure. Wild animal populations show that nonlethal levels of chemical exposure can result in impairment of, or even incapability of reproducing. There are altered animal behaviors in regard to reproduction and aggressiveness that researchers state are likely to be related to alterations of specific nerve pathways by the EDCs.[147]

EDCs Impact on Vertebrate Sexual Development
Japanese Quail

Vertebrates exposed to endocrine disrupting chemicals (EDCs) undergo both short-term and long-term alterations that result in decreased reproduction and fitness. In studying Japanese quail, all EDCs impaired reproduction, regardless of potential mechanism of action. Exposure during fetal development in the uterus to a variety of EDCs results in the impairment of male sexual behavior.[148]

Japanese quail exposed during embryonic development to estrogen or androgen (testosterone) active EDCs between 0 and 4 days, demonstrated that the developing neural system is vulnerable to lifelong alteration in reproductive function.[149]

Researchers who exposed Japanese quail and mice to several EDCs that included DES and bisphenol A during early embryonic development found the chemicals alter the normal sexual differentiation of the adult animals. The chemicals often induced a sex-reversal that resulted in alteration of the sexually differentiated behaviors in the adult animal. The study concluded that: ". . . the data presented here should stimulate a critical reanalysis of the way to determine the 'safe' exposure levels to EDCs for wild species and humans, considering behavior and related neural circuits among the factors to be analyzed."[150] They are making the case that present testing methods for determining the toxicity of EDCs are not adequate to identify the full impact on fetal cellular development and function.

Many studies have now been published that identify that there is a connection between environmental pollution and altered sexual development and fertility. Researchers seeing the importance of identifying the chemicals and their potentially harmful effects concluded their 2009 study published in *Reviews of Environmental Contamination & Toxicology* with the appeal:

"We, herewith, make a plea for long-term studies to monitor effects of various environmental chemicals on wildlife vertebrate populations. Such studies may be augmented or combined with mechanistically-oriented histological, cytological, and biochemical parallel investigations, to fill knowledge gaps."[151]

These pleas for studies focused on the full effects of EDCs are becoming more and more imperative when interference in regards to disruption of sexual development, including sex-reversal, is increasingly showing up in the published studies.

The conclusions from the studies make it important to ask the question:

Could the estrogenic and anti-testosterone effects of sunscreens affect the male and female differentiation that needs to take place in order for the developing human fetus to mature into normal adult sexual behavior?

Since fish develop mixed male and female reproductive organs and birds are showing impairment of male sexual behavior including sex-reversal on exposure to EDCs, then disruption of the male and female brain differentiation during human fetal development in the uterus is a very real possibility. This has enormous implications and should not continue to be ignored. There is no way of identifying the outcome of the estrogenic influence of EDC sunscreens during the critical time of fetal brain development, when male brains need to be bathed in testosterone for normal gender differentiation into maleness and male sexual behavior.

EDCs Impact on Human Reproductive Organ Development

Could the reproductive organ changes seen in male fish appear in human males?

Human Male Reproductive Organ Disorders

The studies on fish presented earlier clearly show male reproductive organ disorders, low sperm counts, and sperm of low quality, as demonstrated by their lack of normal functioning. In deciding if humans could be affected by sunscreen chemicals, we can look at whether there are similarities in the human male adult population compared to what has been found in the fish that are exposed to the sunscreen UV filters.

Studies on men in Europe over the last several decades are identifying increasing incidence of male reproductive organ problems. A 1992 *British Medical Journal* (BMJ) article concluded with the concern:

"There has been a genuine decline in semen quality over the past 50 years. As male fertility is to some extent correlated with sperm count the results may reflect an overall reduction in male fertility. The biological significance of these changes is emphasized by a concomitant increase in the incidence of genitourinary abnormalities such as testicular cancer and possibly also cryptorchidism (undescended testicles) and hypospadias (male urethra opening on underside of penis), suggesting a growing impact of factors with serious effects on male gonadal function."[152]

Researchers have identified that normal male androgen (testosterone) action is critical for the proper development of the penis, as well as for the testicles to descend properly. When estrogens interfere with normal development, both undescended testicles (cryptorchidism) and unusually placed openings on the penis (hypospadias) can occur. Environmental endocrine disruptors can alter the estrogen-androgen ratio as well as act as hormone mimics (either increasing or decreasing their effects), which can result in abnormal development of male reproductive organs.[153] Since ethically, human subjects cannot be used for researching these affects directly, we must rely on experimental data that is available from animal and fish studies. Changes in fish and animal reproduction, combined with the biochemical reasonableness that hormonally active chemicals would impact male reproductive development, provides a realistic hypothesis that if these chemicals are causing the changes in reproductive structures and function in fish and animals; then these chemicals are also of high risk for creating undesirable changes to human reproductive development and health.

Cryptorchidism: Undescended Testicles

The incidence of undescended testicles has been steadily rising over the last few decades. There are differences in incidence rates around the world, depending on the country. Nigeria where sunscreen is difficult to obtain and is not needed due to the natural protection of the melanin in black skin, a study published in 2001 established their rate for cryptorchidism at less than 1%.[154]

In the United States, the prevalence of cryptorchidism is 3.7% at birth. Internationally, prevalence ranges from 4.3 to 4.9% at birth.[155] A study published in 2004 showed the rate in Denmark is significantly higher than what was reported 40 years ago, with an incidence rate at birth of 9.0%. They also determined that the incidence rate was 2.4% in Finland. The authors stated that the higher prevalence of congenital cryptorchidism in Denmark compared to Finland correlates with the pattern also seen in Danish men who have a high frequency of reproductive problems, testicular cancer, and impaired semen quality. They theorized that this is most likely explained by environmental factors, which includes endocrine disrupters (EDCs) and lifestyle.[156]

Japanese researchers identified a specific recessive gene that could be interacting with estrogenic environmental EDCs that is resulting in cryptorchidism for a percentage of the newborns.[157] Other researchers, however, found little correlation for a genetic cause of these abnormalities. With the recognition that testosterone is essential for the descent of the testicles before birth, and that the incidence rates have risen so rapidly, they concluded that environmental factors may have a role, and stated environmental interactions and their affect on genes need to be studied to identify what is behind the increasing rate of cryptorchidism.[158]

Hypospadias: Abnormally Placed Urethral Opening on Penis

Hypospadias is one of the most common congenital disorders in males. In this disorder, the opening of the urethra occurs on the underside of the penis, or on the perineum, rather than at the tip. At this time there is a lack of agreement as to whether the incidence of this malformation is increasing. The researchers, themselves, say part of the problem is the difficulty in creating standardized and objective assessment guidelines.[159]

When considering the cause of hypospadias, several findings are worth further investigation. Since sunscreens function like estrogens, anti-estrogens, and anti-androgens, they are capable of causing disruption in the process of male reproductive organ development.

Hypospadias: Incidence Rates Differ with Race

In a study designed to identify the possible factors influencing the occurrence of hypospadias, researchers in Washington State found increased risk for this condition to be associated with 3 factors: White race; older age birth mothers; and preexisting diabetes in the mothers.[160]

In California, a study looking at births from 1984 through 1997 also found maternal White race to be associated with increased risks for hypospadias.[161] A later study looking at California births from 1997 through 2000 identified that both Black and White races were associated with a higher risk of hypospadias compared to the Hispanic race.[162]

There is clear agreement that androgens (male hormones) are critical for proper penile development. Researchers have also determined if the natural male hormone action on the fetus is impaired, there is disruption in the masculinization of the fetus, including the formation of the external genitalia, which can result in this abnormality.[163]

Higher Levels of: Sunscreens in Whites and Pesticides in Blacks
Hypospadias has a greater incidence rate for children and grandchildren born to women who took the estrogenic DES during pregnancy. The study above identifies higher incidence rates in both Blacks and Whites. The concentrations of estrogenic sunscreen chemicals are higher in Whites, and estrogenic pesticides are higher in Blacks. Based on these factors, it is reasonable to suspect the presence of sunscreen chemicals, as well as pesticides could be associated with this increasing male reproductive disorder that is being seen in several countries around the world. More research needs to be directed toward determining whether sunscreen chemicals are involved in hypospadias development.

In looking into whether hypospadias could be caused by brominated flame retardants or PCBs, which are now so prevalent, one study found no association between the incidence of this malformation and levels of these chemicals in the mother's blood.[164] Research is still ongoing and no absolute conclusions as to the cause have been determined.

Testicular Cancer on the Rise
Testicular cancer is a growing problem, mainly in highly developed industrialized countries. In the U.S., White males under 50 years had an incidence rate of testicular cancer of 4.1 per 100,000 in 1973. By 1999, the incidence rate had almost doubled to 8.0 per 100,000. During this time, the Black incidence was less than 1 per 100,000, which over the 26 years increased only to 1.6 per 100,000 by 1999.[165]
The most common type of adult testicular cancer has been determined to have its origins during fetal development in the uterus. These adult cancers are arising from cells that were formed in the embryo before birth, and caused by a disturbed process of cellular migration or organization.[166] The primary event is the arrest of germ-cell differentiation caused by testicular dysgenesis (abnormal fetal development), followed by malignant transformation and overt

cancer after puberty in young adults. Researchers have concluded that environmental factors, including maternal lifestyle and possibly an early exposure to EDCs, combined with individual genetic susceptibility, are the primary causes.[167]

Studies carried out in the Danish population have determined that the risk of testicular cancer in first-generation immigrants to Denmark was lower than the risk seen in native-born Danes. The numbers also reflected that the risk in second-generation immigrants was similar to that found in Denmark natives. These findings make the case for a substantial influence of environmental factors limited to the period early in life, most probably to the period when the fetus is developing in the uterus.[168]

In 2010, a doctor examining the available evidence regarding the clustering of the conditions of poor semen quality, hypospadias, cryptorchidism, and testicular cancer that has been seen increasing throughout the 20th and into the 21st century, concluded that the origins remain unclear, endocrine disruptors cannot explain it all, but could involve a multi-generational process of environmental origin that creates genetic damage in the egg and sperm cells.[169]

Male Infertility on the Rise

One researcher stating that biologists working with wildlife have been concerned about the possible effects of endocrine disrupting chemical agents on animal reproduction, but there has been less concern about detrimental effects in humans. He states that exposure to endocrine disrupters needs to be addressed as there is an increasing incidence of hormone-dependent cancers (e.g., breast, prostate, testicular), and increasing incidence of male reproductive health problems (hypospadias, undescended testis, poor semen quality) that are symptoms of an underlying testicular dysgenesis syndrome. Fertility problems are now so common that assisted reproduction is necessary for 5% of all children born in Denmark. He claims that both experimental and epidemiological studies provide evidence that points toward the increasing incidence of these conditions as being the result of disruption of normal fetal programming and reproductive organ development due to adverse environmental effects during pregnancy, making EDCs a possibility.[170]

In addition to EDCs having the ability to lead to abnormal fetal development, increasing ROS could also be contributing to declining sperm quality. When ROS cannot be balanced by the body's antioxidant level, the resultant oxidative stress has been considered a major contributory factor to infertility, as it leads to sperm damage and deformity, eventually resulting in male infertility.[171] In examining causes of the oxidative stress that is leading to abnormal sperm function, one study included aging, and environmental toxicants (e.g., EDCs) as likely to induce the oxidative stress.[172]

Semen Quality Reduced

Researchers in Paris followed 1,351 healthy fertile men for the 20 year period from 1973 to 1992. They determined that the concentration and motility of sperm and the percentage of morphologically normal spermatozoa declined over the study period, a decline that was not found to be related to the age of the men.[173]

November 29, 2010 – *Internal Medicine News*
European Science Foundation Sounds Alarm on Male Infertility

A report by the European Science Foundation (ESF) published in *Internal Medicine News* highlights the enormity of the male infertility problem. In it, they warned that too little attention and money are being spent looking into the problem of lower fertility rates in men in Europe. This report written by a high level group of Europe's leading experts from 79 research institutions cites that in Europe there is a growing demand for assisted fertilization techniques. They claim evidence points towards adverse trends in male reproductive health, including reduced semen quality, increased incidence of testicular cancer and increased or an already high incidence of the congenital reproductive malformations of cryptorchidism and hypospadias.[174]

Sperm counts across Europe have long been reported to be dropping, possibly because of environmental factors. They find that 20% of European men ages 18 to 25 years old have low sperm count (oligospermia). A normal count is 50 to 500 million sperm per ejaculate. Oligospermia is defined as less than 20 million per ejaculate, which leads to infertility problems.[175]

Research into the possibility that it is mutations that could be responsible for the increased male infertility found mutations to be very rare. The article stated that the rapid increase in male reproductive disorders indicates environmental factors or changes in lifestyle rather than genetic factors. Therefore these disorders are intrinsically preventable, provided that the cause or causes can be identified. The corresponding author, Dr. Niels E. Skakkebaek of the University of Copenhagen, of the ESF report mentioned above, voicing the need to increase attention to male reproductive problems, has focused on mothers' exposure to environmental chemicals such as EDCs during pregnancy as being the threat to fetal male reproductive development, creating testicular abnormalities that are frequently precursors to poor fertility.

This same report conveys there is growing evidence that poor male reproductive health is also linked to obesity. In addition, they are identifying a substantial increase in cardiovascular, endocrine, and metabolic diseases in men that may be due to abnormal testosterone levels. The group recommended that a multinational, multidisciplinary research project be funded over the next decade to examine environmental chemicals and genetic background factors affecting male reproductive fitness.[176]

This correlation that low sperm quality may be just a symptom of a larger health picture was also identified by other researchers. A large study of approximately 40,000 men over 40 years found that increasing semen quality was associated with living longer, leading these researchers to hypothesize that good semen quality may be a general biomarker of overall good health.[177] Given that early exposure may impact life-long health, it is important that chemicals that disrupt normal fetal development need to be reassessed as to their safety, which must include the chemicals utilized in sunscreens.

Could Sunscreens Affect Puberty?

Since sunscreens exert an estrogenic influence, it is possible that sunscreens could affect the timing of reproductive development in children. Recognition of the impact of these chemicals is beginning to be addressed as a doctor from Canada writes:

"A more hidden but insidious cause of early puberty is the many environmental toxins, which act as hormone-disruptors. For example, the U.S. Food and Drug Administration only regulates products that contain prescription quantities of the female sex-hormone estrogen. Products containing lower amounts of estrogens – less than 10,000 International Units per ounce – are unregulated. Yet these products do have active feminizing effects on people." "And the number of products that contain estrogen-like chemicals is growing: sunscreens, nail polish, plastic toys and baby bottles, pesticides, shampoos and hair straighteners, meat additives and fillings in teeth. A new term is now current in research literature: HCPs, hormone-containing products."[178]

Indeed, the sunscreens and pesticides this doctor talks about are found in young girls. A study on urine samples looking for estrogenic acting phenol type compounds found BPA, the benzophenone BP3, and the pesticide 2,5-dichlorophenol (25DCP) in more than 94% of the samples collected from girls age 6 to 8. The sunscreen BP3 was found to be the highest, and highest in Whites, as well as highest in the summer. The pesticide 25DCP was found to be higher in Blacks.[179] The scientific community cannot continue to deflect findings like these and continue to tell us that more studies must be conducted before there can be a call to take these chemicals off the market.

What Impact Do EDCs Have on Adult Males?
EDCs Block Testosterone Production and Activity

Since testosterone production is disrupted by sunscreen chemicals, then we need to look at what types of outcomes would be occurring in males who are exposed to them. One sign of excess estrogen in relation to testosterone is male breast enlargement. Statistics state that 2/3 of prepubescent boys and 1/2 of adult men have breast enlargement. It is well established that drugs can create this condition. Some of the known ones are: the stomach acid drug (Tagamet); the heart drug (Aldactone); and the anti-androgen prostate cancer drug (Casodex). Since some of the sunscreen chemicals act like estrogens and some act stronger than prostate cancer anti-androgen drugs, sunscreens would also have the potential of causing male breast enlargement.[180]

Increased Breast Reduction Surgeries in Males

The U.S. has seen a large increase in the number of male breast reduction surgeries, which could be an indicator as to whether the incidence male breast enlargement is increasing. In February 2010 a British news media reported: "Plastic surgeons are reporting a record number of 'man boob' reduction operations as the rise in demand outstrips that for all other procedures – including women's breast enlargement." The British Association of Aesthetic Plastic Surgeons (BAAPs) who represent about one third of Britain's plastic surgeons reported that in 2009 breast reduction surgeries in men grew by 80%, when male cosmetic surgery overall grew by only 21%.[181]

World-wide statistics show there are quite a number of these surgeries performed as shown below.[182]

2009 – World-wide Gynecomastia Surgery

U.S.	49,932
Brazil	33,575
China	32,343
India	24,720
Japan	10,943
South Korea	9,718
Mexico	7,970
Germany	6,429
Turkey	5,999
Italy	5,250
Britain	4,359
France	4,060
Russia	4,007
Spain	3,515
Taiwan	2,747
Colombia	2,518
Venezuela	2,086
Thailand	2,017
Argentina	1,928
Canada	1,785
Portugal	1,750
Australia	1,736
Belgium	1,724
Saudi Arabia	1,720
Hungary	1,148
Others	27,005
TOTAL	250,984

It appears that the increasing number of estrogenic EDCs is contributing to this male breast enlargement problem. These numbers only represent the men who are bothered enough to seek out surgery. How many young boys and men do you see every day with this problem that appears to be increasing around the world as demonstrated by the above statistics?

Could Sunscreen Chemicals Be Affecting Adult Females?
Breast Cancer

Hormone dependent cancers are found in higher incidence among the affluent countries leading some researchers to state the most plausible explanation is a high protein and high fat diet. However, one thing that affluent countries have in common is the number of estrogenic chemicals that are produced and utilized, including sunscreens. Since sunscreens disrupt normal female and male hormones balances, then cancers that are sensitive to these hormones would be more common where they are used.

Breast Cancer Cell Line Experiments

Researchers use breast cancer cells in the laboratory to test whether a chemical is estrogenic or not. When a chemical is estrogenic, it causes increased cell division to occur in the cultured breast cancer cells.

An organization called Zero Breast Cancer has been involved in a research project to determine environmental effects on breast tissue, which has identified the phenol bisphenol A (BPA) shows increased breast cell growth, as well as the development of cancerous lesions in mice. Prenatal exposure from the mother passes this effect through to the offspring of rats. Their Website cites research results of several studies that identify exposure to BPA during fetal development permanently alters the normal development of the mammary (breast) gland making the fetus more susceptible to environmental hormones than the adult due to irreversible effects that occur that affect organ development. One of the articles ended with the conclusion: "These findings strengthen the hypothesis that exposure to xenoestrogens (e.g., BPA, sunscreen chemicals) during early development may be an underlying cause of the increased incidence of breast cancer observed in European and U.S. human populations over the last 50 years."[183]

Since the benzophenones that are used as UVB sunscreens are part of the same phenol chemical family, we need to assume they could have the same affect on humans until proven otherwise. A group of researchers published studies in 2001 and 2004 that tested sunscreen chemicals to determine if they act estrogenically on breast cancer cells. Out of the 9 sunscreen chemicals they tested, they found 8 to be estrogenic, as they increased breast cancer cell division. Table 9 below illustrates their reported findings.[184]

Table 9. **Breast Cancer Cell Division by Sunscreen Chemicals**

Chemicals Tested	2001 Reported Results	2004 Reported Results
Benzophenones		
BP1	Not Tested	Yes
BP2	Not Tested	Yes
BP3	Yes	Yes
Salicylate		
Homosalate HMS	Yes	Yes
Camphors		
3-BC	Not Tested	Yes
4-MBC	Yes	Yes
Cinnamate		
OMC	Yes	Yes
PABA		
OD-PABA	Yes	Yes
Avobenzone	No	No

Table 9. Sunscreen chemicals BP1, BP2, BP3, HMS, 3-BC, 4-MBC, OMC, OD-PABA create cell division in breast cancer cells. Avobenzone showed no reaction.

Avobenzone

The results from these studies indicate that avobenzone may not be estrogenic as it does not increase the division of breast cancer cells, however, there are concerns over its safety. Avobenzone has been incorporated into sunscreens for protection from UVA radiation. The studies that have been performed so far on avobenzone have mostly only looked into whether they create an allergic contact reaction on the skin, and how much they cover of the UV radiation range. As of the date of this writing, very few studies appear on a PubMed search (US National Library of Medicine of over 19 million citations from life science journals) in regards to the potential for estrogenic activity of this new sunscreen.[185]

The few studies that have been published demonstrated that researchers using human volunteers found that avobenzone, as well as the cinnamate EHMC, significantly penetrate through the epidermis of the skin.[186] In examining whether it offers protection, researchers confirmed previous results that it not only did not protect skin cells from the UVA rays, it increased the oxidative effects, and led to significant cell death, as well as decreased the body's natural protective effects of antioxidants.[187]

Oxybenzone BP3

Another study demonstrated the compounds that oxybenzone metabolizes into act as estrogens and increase breast cancer cell growth. The amount of growth depends on which metabolite is formed, as well as the concentration level it attains. The metabolites acted stronger than the strongest human estrogen, estradiol (E2). It is unclear as to what happens when sunscreens cross through human skin and get inside our tissues and organs. Once the sunscreens are in the human body, there is no way of knowing what metabolites they are transforming into or what concentration levels they will attain.[188]

These experiments on breast cancer cells show that the common ingredients found in sunscreens are estrogenic and do have the potential to increase cancer risk throughout the body, not just in the skin.

Sunscreens Impact on Body-wide Fetal Development
Disrupted Bone Formation

The ability of bone forming cells in rats to divide and grow is decreased in the presence of BP3, as well as bisphenol A (BPA). This cytotoxic effect means sunscreens could, in addition to decreasing vitamin D directly, decrease new bone cell formation, which would result in all the conditions connected with weak bones (e.g., osteoporosis, rickets).[189]

Thyroid Disrupting Chemicals (TDCs)

Researchers investigating the endocrine disrupting chemicals (EDCs) have identified that they have the potential for disruption to thyroid hormones also, which is just as important to investigate, and as a result have termed the chemicals that interfere with thyroid function as thyroid disrupting chemicals or TDCs.

The thyroid gland and the hormones it secretes govern the body's basic metabolism. Its major hormones are thyroxine (T4) and triiodothyronine (T3). Normal levels are so crucial for the health of the entire body, T4 and T3 are monitored as part of routine medical physical check-ups.

Benzophenones
BP2

Research on rats has identified that BP2 acts as a TDC. It disrupts the functioning of thyroid hormones by inhibiting the enzyme thyroid peroxidase (TPO), which is necessary for the production of T4 and T3. The rats had significantly decreased T4 hormone. They also had significantly increased thyroid stimulating hormone (TSH), which the body naturally increases in its attempts to raise the level of the crucially important T4 hormone. After only 5 days of treatment with BP2, the rats exhibited hormonal changes characteristic of the beginnings of a hypothyroid state, showing the strong anti-thyroid potential of BP2. This effect did not occur when iodine was added, but was even more pronounced in the absence of iodide. The authors expressed their concern, concluding that: "This new challenge for endocrine regulation must be considered in the context of a still prevailing iodide deficiency in many parts of the world."[190]

BP2 Acts Like a TDC on Rat Thyroid Metabolism

Decreased thyroid peroxidase (TPO)
Decreased T4
Increased thyroid stimulating hormone (TSH)

Cinnamates

Octyl-methoxycinnamate (OMC)

Since octyl-methoxycinnamate (OMC) has been investigated for estrogenic activity, researchers examined the affect it would have on the function of the body's interacting endocrine glands, the hypothalamo-pituitary-thyroid (HPT) axis, due to the fact that estrogen receptors are throughout the entire axis. Rats were given either the human ovarian estrogenic hormone, estradiol (E2), or varying doses of OMC for 5 days. The OMC rats had decreased thyroid hormone that led to interference in the entire interdependent axis of the hypothalamus, pituitary, and thyroid glands. The lowered thyroid hormone levels do not provide the feedback response the other hormone producing glands require for their normal functioning. This has serious implications as the proper functioning thyroid hormones are essential for the basic metabolism and energy of the body.[191]

TDCs Impact Fetal Development

TDCs are of major concern for public health issues as normal thyroid hormone levels are also essential for the proper development of the fetal nervous system and brain, from the time of early conception, throughout the gestation, as well as during early child development. TDCs are capable of creating a disruption of the proper signaling of thyroid hormones in the developing human brain, which can result in permanent alterations and deficits in mental development.[192] Depressed thyroid hormones due to the use of sunscreens that contain BP2 and OMC could have serious adverse affects on fetal development throughout pregnancy.

Autism

Considering all the aspects of impact that sunscreen chemicals have on the developing fetus, and all the features that autistic children display, it is important to pay attention to the correlations that appear between these two. From a biochemical point of view, there are a number of reasons to explore the possibility of a connection between sunscreen chemicals and autism.

Has there been an increase in autism rates that has followed the inception of the widespread use of sunscreens? In the 1970s in the U.S., England, Japan, Sweden and Canada, autism was called childhood schizophrenia. The incidence rate in the U.S. at that time was between 3.1–4.5 in 10,000, or only 1 in 2,222. The U.S. Centers for Disease Control *Morbidity and Mortality Weekly Report* (MMWR) showed a 57% increase in prevalence between 2002 and 2006. In 2002, the average incidence was 6 per 1,000, which climbed to 9.4 per 1,000 in 2006. The increase was higher in boys who showed an incidence of 9.5 per 1,000 in 2002, climbing to 15.2 per 1,000 in 2006, a 60% increase. Girls incidence rate was 2.3 per 1,000 in 2002, a number that also rose to 3.4 per 1,000 by 2006, a 48% increase. These numbers mean that the prevalence climbed staggeringly to 1 in 110, with 1 in 70 boys affected compared to 1 in 315 females.[193]

It has not stopped rising. Just two short years later, in 2009, the number climbed to 1 in 91, with still more boys affected as the number in boys rose to 1 in 58.[194] Researchers state this fast a change has to be from environmental factors, rather than genetic. Environment also deserves attention because even though these figures have kept climbing, the Amish today still only have an incidence rate of 1 in 10,000.[195]

The features of autism that make it important to look into chemical sunscreens' potential role in the rapid increase in autism include:

1. Gender differences
2. Thyroid disruption
3. Hormone disruption
4. Racial differences
5. Rise in incidence parallels rise in sunscreen use

1. Gender differences:

Since most sunscreen chemicals act like estrogens or as anti-androgens, disrupting testosterone, there would be more impact on male development compared to female. One researcher suggests that BPA should be looked into as a possible agent that is exposing the fetus and children to estrogenic developmental disruption. He states it deserves further study due to the fact that autism affects boys to girls in a 4:1 ratio, and BPA acts like an estrogen.[196] He focused on the BPA, but all EDCs that act like estrogens need to be investigated, and this includes the sunscreen chemicals.

As stated earlier in this book, sunscreen chemicals exert many hormonal influences including being estrogenic. Sunscreens do appear to be a difference in influence between boys and girls as evidenced by their differences in birth weights when mothers are identified with sunscreen chemicals in their blood.

Since sunscreen chemicals disrupt sexual development in fish and birds, then there is the possibility of disrupted sexual development in humans. When studying individuals who are transgender, researchers found that transmen (female to male) had higher scores for autistic traits compared with typical males and females.[197]

2. Thyroid disruption:

The human embryo is "exquisitely sensitive" to thyroid disruption during development, and environmental contaminates within the uterus can interfere with its normal process.[198] A researcher looking at the effect of the toxins PCBs and dioxins on the thyroid during fetal development found that the brain is very susceptible to disruption from these toxins. He stated: "It is possible that transient exposure of the mother to doses of toxins presently considered nontoxic to the mother could have an impact upon fetal or perinatal neurological development. If the toxins act via their effect on thyroid hormone action, it is possible that doses of toxins that would normally not alter fetal development, could become deleterious if superimposed on a pre-existing maternal/ or fetal thyroid disorder."[199]

As detailed earlier in this book, sunscreen chemicals disrupt fetal thyroid development in mammals, and autism is being linked to thyroid deficiencies, particularly during fetal development. Studies that examine environmental anti-thyroid chemicals are being called to be performed.[200] Abnormal thyroid function affects development of speech and cognitive skills, both of which are disrupted in the autism spectrum. One study states that: "... it is possible that impaired thyroid function is a cause of some of the symptoms of autism, especially language impairment and mental retardation."[201]

3. Hormone disruption:

Two researchers, identifying that there is little known about the affects of persistent organic pollutants such as PCBs and pesticides, which are endocrine disrupting chemicals the same as sunscreens, on the hormonal balance of the developing brain, urged that research be expanded to include this area. They stated: "It is of particular importance, because doses which are low for adults might become toxic for fetuses, infants or children. Recently, the public concern has been focused on POP (persistent organic pollutants) effects on brain function, concomitantly with the increase in neuropsychiatric disorders, including autism, attention deficit and hyperactivity disorder (ADHD) as well as learning disabilities."[202]

Sunscreen chemicals may just be part of the milieu of synthetic chemicals that mothers now have in their systems. Since the studies are all showing that it is an additive effect of many chemicals, even though each is at a low level, it could be that they are just a part of what is impacting the delicate development of the human brain.

4. Racial differences:

Statistics looking for differences in autism incidence rates have found that there are differences between racial groups. There is a higher incidence of autism in the White race compared to Blacks, Hispanics, and Asians.[203] As stated earlier in the book, the White race has higher concentrations of sunscreen chemicals in their bloodstreams compared with other races.

5. Incidence rise parallels rise in sunscreen use:

In the 1970s and 1980s, the number of children who were diagnosed with autism was around 1 in 2,000. It has been since that time that the incidence has climbed to 1 in 91, which is also the same time period that sunscreens were introduced and then mass marketed, being used by millions.

Based on these connections, it is imperative to research whether the ubiquitous use of sunscreen chemicals, possibly combined with the many other estrogenic chemicals (e.g., pesticides) that have been introduced over the last 30, could be involved in the exponential rise in autism that has also occurred in the last 30 years.

The Fetal Basis of Adult Disease

Obesity and EDCs

Scientists are beginning to recognize that weight may not be the result of excess or wrong calories, but that adult diseases such as obesity may have their origins from alterations that occurred during fetal development. Several factors have become apparent regarding health in our children.

1. The chronic diseases of type 2 diabetes, childhood asthma, attention deficit hyperactivity disorder (ADHD), and obesity are becoming epidemic.
2. Classic gene mutations cannot account for them because the increases have been so large in such a short time.

As a result, a whole new society of investigators has been created called the *International Society for Developmental Origins of Health and Disease* (DOHaD). Finding that environmental interactions altering expression of genes during critical periods of fetal development are playing large roles in the origins of these diseases, researchers have come up with the hypothesis they have termed the developmental basis of health and disease, or "the fetal basis of adult disease".[204]

Researchers investigating obesity have determined that the current obesity epidemic may be the result of the quality of the nutrition of the pregnant mother when she is exposed to environmental chemicals that act like estrogens during crucial times in the development of the fetus. They have recognized that environmental estrogen exposure acting on the genes at critical times alters the pathways involved in food metabolism and changes the "setpoint" or increases susceptibility for obesity later in life. Identifying that exposure to EDCs during fetal development results in alterations in adult metabolism, researchers have come up with the hypothesis they have called: "The Developmental Basis of Obesity." The progression is outlined in Table 10.

Table 10.   **The Developmental Basis of Obesity**

An emerging hypothesis is that the obesity epidemic could be due to the interaction of nutrition and chemical exposures during vulnerable windows in development.

We hypothesize that environmental agents and/or nutrition act during development to:

Alter the pathways responsible for control of adipose tissue development.
Increase the number of fat cells.
Alter food intake and metabolism.
Alter insulin sensitivity and lipid metabolism via effects on pancreas, adipose tissue, liver, GI tract, brain and muscle.

The consequence is alteration of the "setpoint" or sensitivity for developing obesity later in life.

Gene–environment interaction: the focus is on development.

The environment alters gene expression during vulnerable windows in development, resulting in altered epigenetic (modification of gene expression) signals and increased to obesity later in life.

Source: Heindel JJ, vom Saal FS. Role of nutrition and environmental endocrine disrupting chemicals during the perinatal period on the aetiology of obesity. *Mol Cell Endocrinol.* 2009. 304(1-2): 90–96. Epub 2009 Mar 9. Reprinted with permission.

Animal studies demonstrate an increase in obesity in offspring from mothers who are exposed to environmental chemicals showing that it does have a developmental origin. Fetal exposure to endocrine disrupting chemicals creates abnormalities in the balanced control systems required to maintain a normal body weight throughout life. Researchers coined the new word *obesogens* after recognizing that:

". . . environmental endocrine disrupting chemicals can act as 'obesogens' that can permanently derange developing regulatory systems required for body weight homeostasis (equilibrium)."[205]

Another researcher who identified that the estrogenic DES led to increased obesity and increased percentage of fat accumulation also recognized: "It is quite possible that complex events, including exposure to environmental chemicals during development, may be contributing to the obesity epidemic."[206]

Protecting Fetal Development: Better Chance at Controlling Adult Obesity

Scientists state the accumulating amount of evidence points to our needing to focus on prevention, by reducing environmental EDCs, along with better nutrition, before and during pregnancy, rather than attempting to bring weight under control as adults or in our children.

As shown before, studies are demonstrating that very small amounts of EDCs have a much higher toxic impact when they are mixed together. Therefore researchers are recommending that it is better to examine these chemicals in combined mixtures rather than one at a time, as they are so ubiquitous (widespread) that there are now mixtures of many EDCs within our own bodies.[207]

There is much awareness and calls to action about the ever increasing obesity epidemic today. The news is replete with warnings of staggering health care costs arising from the medical conditions obesity creates. With sunscreen chemicals now in almost 100% of the American population, this evidence that endocrine disruption during pregnancy sets us up for obesity later in life requires that action be taken to eliminate EDCs as quickly as possible.

Many of the studies that prove the toxicity to the developing fetus of sunscreen chemicals that were approved in the 1980s and declared as safe for human use were not published until 2010. This means that almost 30 years of detrimental harm has been allowed because gestational toxicity studies were not performed, or if they were, the conclusions stated that more testing had to be performed to confirm the results. When there is evidence reported over the years that demonstrate toxicity, the chemical needs to be removed from the market while the confirmatory studies are conducted rather than what we are now faced with: multi-generations of humans being harmed; and our waters polluted by disrupting hormonally active chemicals.

Chapter 10
Chemical Sunscreens – Impact on Oceans

Coral Reefs

Corals are animals, called polyps, with a round, spherical shape, that secrete calcium carbonate (limestone) by combining calcium with carbon dioxide from the water. The calcium carbonate becomes the hard outer shell creating a home for the coral that grows and eventually builds up into a reef.

Millions of corals from over 500 different species make up a reef, as they land and build on top of ones that have died. Coral is a great example of symbiosis. Algae lives inside the sac of each coral polyp providing it with oxygen and nutrients for the coral polyp's survival, while the polyps provide the algae with the carbon dioxide it needs for photosynthesis. Photosynthesis is a process that uses the energy of sunlight to make carbohydrates out of carbon dioxide and water. Therefore, sunlight is the indispensable ingredient for the building of the coral reefs, as photosynthesis is necessary for the symbiotic growth of the reef. This is why coral are only able to exist in shallow water that needs to be very clear, allowing sunlight through, so they grow close to the surface to a maximum depth of 120 feet. They also need salt water and a water temperature between 77–88°F (25–31°C). When sunlight is blocked for any reason, photosynthesis cannot take place, the algae die and consequently the coral dies also. Since disruption to one, leads to disruption of all, coral reefs are a delicately balanced web of life, with each life form dependent on the others.

Coral Bleaching (Coral Death)

There has been a lot of concern over the amount of coral reef bleaching that has taken place over the last several decades. The algae are what are responsible for the magnificent colors that coral reefs display. Since algae are what contribute to the color of coral, scientists state the most obvious sign of sick coral is the bleaching out of its color, caused by the algae either dying or leaving. The coral polyps, in turn, die as they are dependent on the oxygen from the algae to survive. The 1980s have been identified as the period when this loss of color became dramatically worse.[208] The 1980s are also the years when sunscreen use was beginning to be heavily promoted.

The first coral bleaching event occurred in 1979, with 6 major events since then. These include the 1998 El Niño recorded historic highest tropical sea surface temperatures, a year that an estimated 16% of the world's coral became bleached. Also, the 2005 hurricane season in the Caribbean is identified as a year of increased coral bleaching there.[209]

There has been a cyclical change in global temperature that led to a slight warming of the ocean temperature. This rise in temperature occurred mainly within the layer of seawater that starts 800 yards below the surface. Between 1996 and 2010, measurements showed an average rise in seawater temperatures of 0.64°F (0.36°C) above normal.[210] The warmest global ocean temperature was for the year 1997 when it was 1.04°F (0.58°C) above the 20th Century average of 60.4°F (15.7°C). The year 2009 saw an increase of 0.97°F (0.54°C) above the 20th Century average, or an average global ocean temperature throughout the year of 61.4°F (16.2°C).[211]

In the winter of 2010-2011, the ocean waters in the Florida keys reached such record lows that the extreme cold temperatures also led to coral bleaching. The chilling winter brought two weeks of record cold tempertures that were below 50°F (10°C), which created a stress that corals could not survive.[212]

Environmental Impact on Coral Reefs

Experts state that changing ocean temperatures are just one of the increasing numbers of environmental stresses faced by coral reefs around the world.[213] Part of problem seen today is due to population pressure. Near the coasts, the increased population leads to many pollutants from fertilizers, pesticides, and human waste being washed into the waters. All these encourage the growth of algae that can overwhelm and smother the coral. Deforestation of the land can lead to silt entering the water that blocks the vital sunlight the corals require. Without the sun, the algae cannot perform photosynthesis and it dies.[214]

The fish that are caught for eating are part of the coral ecosystem and when they are overfished, harmful predators move in and upset the balance. Researchers have determined that direct contact of coral with 40–70% of the common seaweeds causes a rapid bleaching and death of coral tissue. If there is a balance between seaweed and the herbivores that eat it, keeping the amount of seaweed in check, then coral reefs can thrive. Where there is overfishing of the herbivores, seaweed overgrows, resulting in coral death that shows up as coral bleaching.[215]

In looking at the effects of poor water quality due to run off from population pressures on the corals of the Great Barrier Reef, scientists have determined that it does play an additional role of a lowering of the corals' thermal tolerance, causing the coral to be more susceptible to bleaching with a change in temperature.[216]

Coral Harbor Bacteria

Vibrio Infections

The infections that are caused by *Vibrio* bacteria are far ranging. In humans, species of *Vibrio* cause cholera. Foodborne illness is caused by consumption of shellfish that are contaminated with non-cholera *Vibrio* strains of bacteria.[217] Studies of corals show that they are reservoirs of potentially virulent strains of *Vibrios*. The *Vibrio alginolyticus, V. harveyi* and *V. coralliilyticus* are dominant in the mucus of Brazilian corals and may be a normal component of the coral community habitat.[218]

Bacteria Products Inhibit Algae Photosynthesis

Studies looking at the affects of *Vibrio shilonii* demonstrate the bacteria attach to coral mucus, and then penetrate the outer layer of the coral, where they multiply rapidly.[219] The toxin it produces inhibits the symbiotic algae from its ability to perform photosynthesis, thus it dies.[220] For this reason, the bacteria *Vibrio shilonii* can lead to coral bleaching.[221]

The Pacific Atoll Palmyra: 2009 Bleaching Event

In looking at many variable factors that could be responsible for coral bleaching, researchers at the Pacific Ocean atoll, Palmyra, found even though an increase in temperature appeared to trigger and contribute to bleaching, there was great variability around the reef in the amount of bleaching.

Areas of Higher Water Temperatures Had the Least Bleaching

They identified the opposite of what would be expected if it was increased water temperature alone that caused the bleaching. They found the least amount of bleaching occurred in areas that had higher temperatures and greater temperature variability.

Turbidity Strongest Overall Predictor of Bleaching

The greatest amount of bleaching occurred in the regions of the atoll that had low water visibility due to increased sand cover. In observing this outcome, they determined that turbidity (low visibility) in the water creating lack of the sunlight the algae need was the primary factor and strongest overall predictor for the amount of bleaching.

The researchers also concluded that a large amount of the variability in the bleaching remained unexplained. One of their hypotheses was that the variation is due to micro-habitat differences in environmental conditions.[222]

Australia: Great Barrier Reef

A 2½ year study of a reef off of an island in the Great Barrier Reef found there were extended periods when the daily average water temperatures exceeded the previous 10-year average by more than 1.8°F (1.0°C). In January and February 2002, a bleaching period led to a 64% decrease in algae, followed by recovery to pre-bleaching levels when the water cooled down.

Vibrio bacteria were identified to increase with the increasing temperature that was accompanied by bleaching of the coral colonies. Researchers could not determine if the increase in the *Vibrio* was due to a bacterial infection of the coral, or whether the *Vibrio* multiply as an opportunistic response to a coral host experiencing compromised health.[223]

In 1998, 2002, and 2006, major bleaching events occurred in the Great Barrier Reef that resulted in 21%–40% offshore and approximately 70% inshore corals being affected. Most recovered well, but about 5% of the area suffered high mortality (death), losing between 30–70% of the corals.[224]

The tourism that started on the Great Barrier Reef in the early 1970s prompted the Australian government to declare it a National Marine Park in 1975, with a primary goal of managing human use. These bleaching events occurred after the years that tourism began mushrooming exponentially in the 1980s and 1990s. During this time tourism increased about 30% per year; escalating numbers that made it difficult to control the permits designed to regulate its use.[225]

Chemical UVB Filters Create Coral Bleaching

"Coral reefs are now multi-million dollar recreational destinations and the Great Barrier Reef is an important part of Australia's economy."[226]   In 2010, approximately 2,000,000 visitors explored the Great Barrier Reef.[227]   What effect could sunscreens have in our oceans of the world that millions of people are swimming in daily after they have slathered themselves with sunscreens?

Just as the stress of increased ocean temperatures cause bacteria to proliferate, killing off the algae that the coral polyps' survival depend upon; sunscreen chemicals cause the same type of habitat stress, as they promote the multiplication of viruses that kill off the algae, which in turn leads to coral death and bleaching.

BP3, OMC, 4-MBC, Butyl Paraben (BP): Cause Bleaching

In a 2008 study published in *Environmental Health Perspectives*, Roberto Danovaro and his team of scientists placed samples of coral from seas and oceans around the world in bags full of virus-free seawater with various types and concentrations of sunscreens and compared them with controls that were also incubated in virus-free seawater. The sunscreen chemicals caused dormant viruses to reproduce until the host algae died, releasing the viruses and spreading the infection to its nearby coral. Within 18–48 hours of exposure to the sunscreen, there was a release of large amounts of coral mucous that is composed of algae and coral tissue. Within 96 hours, the sunscreens caused a loss of the algae's membrane integrity and its photosynthesizing pigments, with a complete bleaching of the hard corals. This occurred with sunscreen quantities as small as only 10 μl/L (microliters/liter). Four of the commonly utilized sunscreen ingredients caused this effect. They were the benzophenone BP3, the cinnamate OMC, the camphor 4-MBC, and the preservative used in sunscreens butyl paraben (BP). The same effects were seen at both low and at high concentrations of sunscreens. The corals that were not exposed to the sunscreens remained healthy.

The sunscreen chemicals that were also tested and had either a minor effect, or no effect on bleaching were octocrylene (OCT), the salicylate EHS, and avobenzone, as well as the solvent propylene glycol (PG).[228]

Can Coral Bleaching Now Be Traced to Increased Tourism and Use of Sunscreens?

Since corals are dependent upon algae and their ability to provide oxygen from its photosynthesis from sunlight, the millions of tourists who are inundating the coral reef waters with sunscreen chemicals on their bodies are killing the algae, which results in the death of the coral in the reefs, as the coral cannot survive without the algae.

Going to where tourism is relatively new we can compare the growth in the numbers of tourists to when the area underwent coral bleaching events. Belize experienced an explosive growth in tourism in the 1990s. Even though other parts of the world experienced coral bleaching in the 1980s during times of increased ocean temperatures, Belize did not have a report of coral bleaching until 1995, when it had its first report of coral bleaching, followed by severe coral bleaching in 1998. Now they report 40% of the Belize reef system has experienced bleaching, with blame being placed on coastal development, overfishing, pollution, climate change, and tourism. All of these environmental impacts could combine to put stress on the reefs, but the fact that Belize now has 850,000 tourists a year, the increased amount of sunscreens they are washing into the waters of the reefs has to be an important part of the bleaching.[229]

Researchers studying Mediterranean coral came to the conclusion: it is environmental stressors that lead to the bleaching events; and the bacteria are just opportunists that multiply due to the coral being compromised. This matches the work showing that the sunscreens create stress on the coral.[230]

In 2010, researchers investigating whether humans are impacting coral reefs directly through localized activities such as snorkeling, kayaking, and fishing, looked at five sites on the northern shore of Moorea in French Polynesia. Before this study, they stated most studies on coral reefs had focused on pollution or global climate change, and little work had been done on the more localized effects of human presence on corals. Their findings determined that the coral site that hosted four times more tourists, with a significantly greater number of people in the water than the other four sites, had significant loss of total coral. Their results demonstrate that human use does impact coral survival.[231]

Danovaro and fellow researchers stated that world-wide there are roughly 10,000 tons of UV filtering sunscreens produced every year. They estimate approximately 25% of the sunscreen ingredients of each application a person puts on is released into the water after 20 minutes of submersion. Based on these figures, the researchers also estimate that approximately 10% of the world's coral reefs are potentially threatened as tourism continues to increase in tropical reef areas. These researchers put forth the idea that sunscreens could act synergistically with pesticides and hydrocarbons, which also can cause coral bleaching, potentially increasing even more the amount of bleaching that is occurring around the world.[232]

The results of these studies clearly indicate sunscreen chemicals can result in coral death. Use of chemical sunscreens must be brought to an end. The natural beauty the tourists spend million of dollars each year to see needs to be protected by the countries that rely on their beautiful coral reefs as an essential part of their economy. The survival of ocean life is also critical for human survival.

Part 3 – The Nanoparticle Generation

Chapter 11
Nanoparticle Toxicity

Nanoparticles (NP), which are defined as less than 100 nanometers (nm), have been approved for use in sunscreens in the U.S. by the FDA since 1999. These tiny particles that are 1/5,000 the size of a human hair are also approved for use in Europe, Australia, and Japan.[233]

Conflicting Results Regarding Toxicity

In a 2007 *Environmental Pollution* article, Swiss scientists described that the ability to measure whether nanoparticles are safe is greatly hampered by the fact that there are only a few quantitative analytical techniques for measuring nanoparticles in natural systems, so there is a severe lack of information about their occurrence in the environment.[234]

Part of the reason for the problem is that the quantum difference in size when titanium dioxide (TiO_2) or zinc oxide (ZnO) are reduced from the parent bulk material to nanometer particles results in equally large changes in the characteristics of their interactions. They have much greater reactivity and therefore exert different biological effects than those seen in their bulk parent material.[235]

In 2010, a group of researchers stated that studies formulated to investigate the health and safety of these nanomaterials are still lacking.[236] In a December 2010 article, another group of researchers acknowledged that standard test methods are not designed for nanoparticles. Genotoxicity (damaging to DNA) testing is still under revision in regards to TiO_2 and ZnO nanomaterials. As a result, they stated that there is still a limited data base on genotoxicity test results with regard to nanomaterials.[237]

However, there are an increasing number of studies that are revealing there are plenty of reasons to be concerned about the pervasive incorporation of nanoparticles into so many personal items, in addition to the sunscreen products. The studies are revealing nanoparticles are potentially toxic not only for humans, but for all livings things that are exposed to them. The researchers in these recently published studies are finding nanoparticles are harmful when larger concentrations are used, and when studies are run over longer periods of time. Toxicity shows up when additional hours or days are added compared to earlier investigations that were of shorter durations.

Impact on Vertebrates Reveals Toxicity

Even though there have been conflicting results regarding toxicity, a recent study that was presented at a scientific meeting resolves the question. At the November 2010 30th Annual Meeting of the *Society of Environmental Toxicology and Chemistry* (SETAC) in New Orleans, investigators presented the results of their research regarding the effect of TiO_2 nanoparticles on the African clawed frog. They found that coexposure of increasing concentrations of TiO_2 nanoparticles of either 5 or 10 nm, along with UV light, led to a significant decrease in the survival of the frog.[238] The sunscreens are designed and marketed to shield and protect the skin against UV light, however, this study reveals that toxicity is created when the TiO_2 nanoparticles are exposed to the UV light, leading to the death of the frogs.

Chapter 12
Nanoparticle – Impact on Aquatic Environment

Impact on Fish

An article published in 2006, years after the world-wide mass marketing of nanoparticles in sunscreens and cosmetics, stated: "However, release of manufactured nanoparticles into the aquatic environment is largely an unknown." After looking at the available literature they concluded that new research methods are required to be able to address the special properties nanomaterials present. In addition, they suggested that a precautionary approach is required when evaluating the new nanomaterials for their risks to the health of the environment.[239]

Researchers reanalyzed the conflicting findings regarding nanoparticle toxicity that result in the impression that high concentrations of copper and zinc are relatively non-toxic to fish. Their reanalysis revealed that the data does indicate ZnO nanoparticles given in daily doses are toxic to the 3 different species of fish: carp; *Nile tilapia*; and guppy. They hypothesized that ZnO toxicity has not yet been demonstrated in rainbow trout or turbot because the studies conducted so far have only exposed the fish to relatively low doses, and there has been no analysis on effects on growth and reproduction. In looking at zinc metabolism and the way the studies are conducted, they state that the possibility for negative effects to arise from chronic exposure to high doses of zinc in the diet cannot be ruled out, as the negative effects would not be easily detected by only monitoring survival and growth over periods of several weeks or even months.[240]

Investigators looking at the possible toxicity of ZnO nanoparticles on the fresh water protozoan, *Tetrahymena thermophila*, found the toxicities of either nano or bulk ZnO did not differ. The ZnO nanoparticles led to 50% of the protozoan dying after 4 hours of exposure. When compared to either bulk or nanoparticle copper oxide (CuO), they determined the ZnO nanoparticles were extremely more toxic than copper oxide.[241]

In 2008, after a review of the existing published studies investigating engineered nanoparticles impact on the aquatic environment, researchers cited that the few studies that have been published reveal nanoparticles, even in low concentrations, exert acute toxicity on the test organism, the *Daphnia magna* (water flea). In addition, they found nanoparticles interacting with coexisting contaminants in the water adhere to them, which leads to an increase in the toxicity of the other chemicals.[242] Also in that same year, British scientists declared that the release of manufactured nanoparticles in large amounts into the natural aquatic environment is of increasing concern.[243]

Differences in toxicity from the sunscreen chemicals can be seen simply due to changes in how the investigators design the study. When a study looks at only 48 hours of exposure, it could report that little affect is seen and the chemicals could be considered safe. However, a study published in 2010 that extended the exposure to 72 hours found TiO_2 nanoparticles resulted in high toxicity. Extending the exposure time even further to 21 days, they found the significantly harmful changes to *Daphnia magna* that are listed below.

Daphnia magna
21 Day Exposure to TiO_2 Nanoparticles

Severe growth retardation
Reproductive defects
Increased mortality
Difficulty eliminating TiO_2 nanoparticles: resulting in significant bodily accumulation

---

Their conclusion: TiO_2 nanoparticles pose risks in aquatic ecosystems to both individual, as well as entire population levels.[244]

Other researchers concerned about the affect on the aquatic environment exposed carp fish to TiO_2 nanoparticles. They found the carp experienced oxidative stress in their liver and impaired ability to breathe through their gills. Their reported findings are shown below.

Carp
Exposure to TiO_2 Nanoparticles

Liver cells
    Oxidative stress
    Decreased antioxidant enzymes
    Cell injury, necrosis and death

Gill vessels and filaments utilized for respiration
    Edema
    Thickening

These investigators concluded: TiO_2 nanoparticles pose a potential risk when they are released into the aquatic environment.[245]

Chapter 13
Nanoparticle – Impact on Humans

Nanoparticle: Skin Penetration
Nanoparticle Skin Penetration Studies Show Conflicting Results

In looking at the ability of TiO_2 or ZnO nanoparticles to penetrate the skin, one group of researchers tested pig skin and found that it did not penetrate. They concluded, therefore, that these nanoparticles are safe to use in cosmetics.[246]

An April 2010 review of the available studies on human safety of nanoparticles concluded that there was little harm in their use. They cited low dermal toxicity, low mucous membrane irritation, low oral toxicity, and no evidence of a carcinogenic potential. They determined that the studies do not show evidence that the nanoparticulate TiO_2 or ZnO are able to be absorbed by the skin. They also identified there is evidence that these substances protect human skin against UV-induced adverse effects, including DNA damage and skin cancer. However, they did state that inhalation studies in rats suggest an increase in the incidence of lung tumors, but reasoned that rather than being the result of the nanoparticles, the tumors were probably due to a lung overload from exposure to high concentrations of inert dust, dismissing the possibility the tumors could have resulted from the nanoparticle exposure. When studies are supposed to be designed so that the one difference is the variable being tested for, in this case nanoparticles, it makes no sense to claim the harm was caused from dust exposure rather than nanoparticle exposure.

These same researchers stated that as "nano" TiO_2 and ZnO studies continue to be published, that concerns of genotoxicity and photogenotoxicity (light induced DNA damage) of the nanoparticles will appear and care will need to be taken in the area of standardizing how the tests are conducted and how they are interpreted. They claim the over 20 years of human use has not seen clinical case reports nor documented adverse events to support a lack of safety of these chemicals used in sunscreen products, therefore the benefits would seem to outweigh any potential risk. They ended the article with: "'Nano' TiO$_2$ and ZnO are safe for human exposure and should be considered as such based on the entire data set."

These investigators warned ". . . assigning potential toxicity based on a single physical characteristic or because the field of nanotoxicology is in its infancy or since 'more research is needed'. . .", could lead to lack of acceptance of these otherwise acceptable materials.[247] However, both these cautionary statements are true and there does need to be concern in using nano materials. The following section will present articles that highlight the harm these tiny particles can inflict.

TiO$_2$ Nanoparticles: Skin Penetration

Researchers state that nanoparticles do not enter intact skin, but how many people have uncompromised skin? The research is not clear what happens to nanosized particles when the skin barrier is compromised. This is often the case when skin is sunburned, chronically photodamaged, exfoliated (as many skin care programs recommend), has cuts or breaks, or affected by common skin diseases like eczema. When exposed to direct sunlight, TiO$_2$ nanoparticles also create ROS that cause DNA damage.[248]

ZnO Nanoparticles: 2011 Study Proves Skin Penetration

The conflicting results of whether nanoparticles are absorbed was resolved in an Australian study of human volunteers of various nationalities where isotopes of either bulk (110 nm) or nanoparticle (19 nm) ZnO was applied to their backs twice a day for 5 days.

Blood and urine were collected from 8 days before the trial to 11 days after the first application. Everyone showed Zn in their blood and urine starting from day 2 and on day 11. Four subjects who were exposed to the nanoparticles were followed for 25 and 40 days with Zn still being detected in their blood. These researchers concluded there were four key findings from their study:

1. Contrary to the dominant view, this study provides unequivocal evidence that Zn from ZnO nanoparticles in sunscreens is absorbed through healthy human skin exposed to sunlight and is detectable in blood and urine.
2. The total amounts of Zn absorbed from sunscreen were small compared with the amounts of Zn normally present in the human body.
3. Particle size and gender determined the levels of absorption. This may be due to differences in skin thickness (female skin generally thinner than male) or other gender-related factors such as skin pH and surface fat content.
4. There is a time lag between sunscreen application and the first detection of tracer isotope Zn in samples. Detection was first detected in blood after the fourth sunscreen application on the second day. This implies that studies with fewer applications, a shorter observation time, or the use of less sensitive methods to detect absorption may not have been able to observe effects.

This study was evaluated and signed off on by the U.S. Environmental Protection Agency (EPA) in March 2011.[249] The harm that is revealed in the recent studies that are outlined in the book needs action taken rather than continuing to allow these products to be approved by government agencies and to be sold to the public.

Coating Nanoparticles

In looking at the potential for skin penetration of nanoparticles, one study found that pig skin that had undergone hair removal displayed significantly deeper skin penetration of TiO_2 nanoparticles coated with alumina/silica/silicon when compared to controls. They found that the coated TiO_2 entered the vacant hair follicles, which are greater than 1 mm below the skin surface, but stated they did not find evidence that they penetrated through the epidermis into the dermis.[250]

The easier ability for coated nanoparticles to enter vacant hair follicles becomes important as coating nanoparticles is an avenue that manufacturers are pursuing to stabilize very unstable chemicals. The UVA filter avobenzone that has been approved in the EU and the U.S. is very unstable in sunlight, so researchers are looking into ways to combine it to make it more stable.

When combined with either TiO_2 or ZnO uncoated nanoparticles, Avobenzone becomes even more unstable in the sunlight and is reduced to less than 1% of its activity. They have determined that coating the TiO_2 nanoparticles with silica retains 76% of its ability to filter sun rays.[251]

This necessity to coat the nanoparticles to make the sunscreen retain any ability to filter sun rays is critically important. In a 2010 *Toxicological Sciences* study researchers, in testing whether coating the nanoparticles would decrease cellular toxicity, found that when TiO_2 nanoparticles are silicone coated, the coating appears to lead to greater toxicity, inducing significant lung inflammation. This study identified the silicone surface coating increases its toxicity rather than making it less harmful.[252]

TiO_2 Nanoparticles: Induce Significant Skin Aging

In a 2009 *Toxicology Letters* article, researchers applying TiO_2 nanoparticles to pig skin samples isolated in the lab found the nanoparticles did not penetrate the skin. However, when they applied it to living pigs' ears for 60 days, they found TiO_2 nanoparticles did penetrate through the skin, and became widely distributed in tissues including the brain and liver, while inducing significant changes in the skin. The skin and liver displayed the most severe pathological lesions due to the oxidative stress that was induced by the deposited nanoparticles. These researchers warned that prolonged use of TiO_2 nanoparticles would lead to significant skin aging as the nanoparticles significantly reduced the collagen content of the skin. They concluded, "Altogether, the present study indicates that nanosize TiO_2 may pose a health risk to humans after dermal (skin) exposure over a relative long time period."[253]

TiO_2 and ZnO Nanoparticles: Generate ROS

Since the UVA rays create more reactive oxygen species (ROS), using the UVA blocking TiO_2 and ZnO nanoparticles appears on the surface to be the answer to stop the potential for damage by ROS. However, both TiO_2 and ZnO nanoparticles, by themselves, generate ROS in the laboratory. It is ROS that created the pathological lesions in the organs of the mice in the *Toxicology Letters* study cited above.

In a 1997 *FASEB Letter* (Federation of American Societies for Experimental Biology), researchers identified that TiO_2 nanoparticles absorb about 70% of UV radiation, which leads to the generation of ROS, which in turn leads to oxidative stress. They demonstrated that sunlight-illuminated TiO_2 creates and accelerates DNA damage both in the laboratory and in human cells. Identifying the toxicity, the investigators stated: "These results may be relevant to the overall effects of sunscreens."[254]

Researchers at the University of California, Los Angeles concluded their 2006 study of nanotechnology by stating: "Although very little is currently known about this area, it is probably wise to regard NM (nanomaterial) waste as potentially hazardous until proven otherwise." ". . . we can no longer postpone safety evaluations of NM.

A proactive approach is required, and the regulatory decisions should follow from there." They also suggested that due to their ability to attach to mitochondria (the energy producing parts of every cell) and to initiate programmed cell death, the toxicity of nanoparticles could be utilized in fighting cancer cells.[255] These actions of nanoparticles should be of concern in regard to healthy cells being exposed to nanoparticles, and any questions regarding their ability to lead to cell death should be completely resolved before use of nanoparticles continues to be promoted and sold in the wide variety of products including cosmetics, body lotions, and soaps as they are today.

A 2009 article published in *Small Journal* demonstrated that TiO_2 nanoparticles create cellular damage due to the impairment of cell function, as the nanoparticles result in:

Decreased cell size
Decreased cell proliferation
Decreased mobility
Decreased ability to contract collagen (the primary protein fiber that provides the framework for the foundational matrix of the body's connective tissue).

They found TiO_2 nanoparticles easily penetrate through the cell membrane while larger particle aggregates of TiO_2 are brought physically into the cell by surrounding them and pulling them inside. When the TiO_2 nanoparticles are inside the cell, they are taken inside vesicles that continue to pull more particles in until the vesicles rupture.

These researchers realizing the importance of protecting cells and tissue from damage, tested polymer coating the nanoparticles and found they had less adherence to the cell membrane, which would decrease their ability to penetrate the cell. This they stated would in turn decrease the generation of reactive oxygen species (ROS) formation, protecting cells, even in the absence of light exposure.[256] Here again, there are conflicting results as others described previously in the book found silicone coating makes TiO_2 more toxic.[257] These conflicts are essential to resolve before continuing to allow products that contain coated nanoparticles to be marketed to the public.

Resolving the Conflicting Results From
Studies on Skin Penetration and Toxicity

Researchers, themselves, explain that the variability in the results of studies examining TiO_2 nanoparticles and their potential for entering the skin, as well as for toxicity potential may be due to the utilization of different types of mammalian cells involved, differing sources of the nanoparticles, as well as variations in the techniques of treatment preparation. Additionally, result data can be misinterpreted because the different physical and chemical properties that nanoparticles display can interfere with the various dyes that are used in the technical assays where results are dependent on color changes.

2010 *Toxicology in Vitro* Study on TiO_2 Nanoparticles

In a 2010 study published in *Toxicology in Vitro*, R.K. Shukla and associates exposed human epidermal skin cells to TiO_2 nanoparticles and tested whether the nanoparticles entered the cells and what effect they had on the skin cells. They chose concentrations of nanoparticles that are far less than those utilized in cosmetics. The highest concentration of TiO_2 nanoparticles they used was 80 micrograms per milliliter (80 µg/mL) or only 0.080 milligrams per milliliter (0.08 mg/mL), far less than even 1 milligram (mg).[258]

Commercial sunscreen concentrations of TiO_2 nanoparticles are between 3–15% of the total volume in a tube/bottle, and the U.S. FDA approval is for up to 25%. Depending on the concentration in the creams or lotions, 5 milliliters (ml) contains between 150–750 mg of nanoparticles, or 100s of times more than the amount utilized in the above study. The researchers claim the lower concentrations are realistic, as this could be the concentration of nanoparticles that are left on the skin even after the lotion is washed off.

Study Reveals TiO₂ Nanoparticles Penetrate Skin, Cells, and Nucleus
The human epidermal skin cells exposed to TiO_2 nanoparticles showed a significant cellular uptake of the nanoparticles that were between 30–100 nm. They penetrated the cell membrane and the membrane of the nucleus, getting not only inside the cell (inside the cytoplasm), but inside the nucleus (DNA containing part of cell) as well. See Figure 6 below.

Human Epidermal Cells with Internalized TiO₂ Nanoparticles

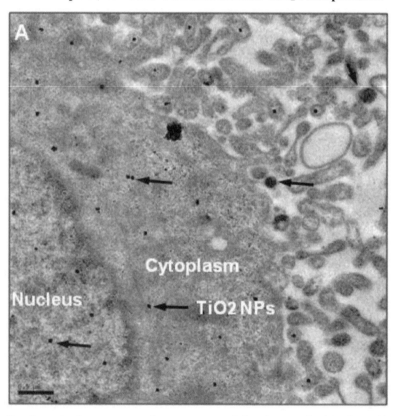

In photo A, the arrows point to nanoparticles that are inside the cell membrane, as well as inside the nucleus of the cell.

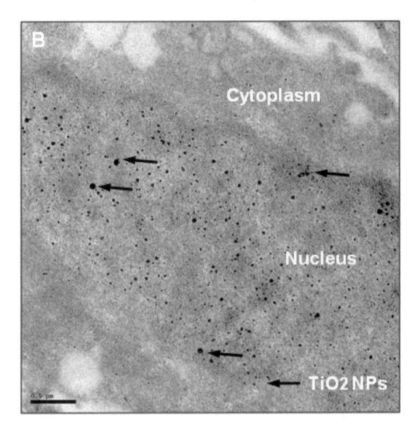

In photo B, a higher powered image of the cell with arrows pointing to the nanoparticles inside the nucleus of the cell.

Figure 6. TEM (transmission electron microscope) photomicrographs of human epidermal cells showing internalization of TiO$_2$ nanoparticles (8 µg/ml) in cytoplasm and nucleus (A-B). Arrows indicate the presence of TiO$_2$ nanoparticles inside different cellular organelles (specialized cell structures).

Source: Shukla RK, Sharma V, Pandey AK, Singh S, Sultana S, Dhawan A. ROS-mediated genotoxicity induced by titanium dioxide nanoparticles in human epidermal cells. *Toxicol in Vitro*. 2011. 25(1):231-241. Epub 2010 Nov 17. Reprinted with permission.

The difference in the potential for toxicity between bulk and nanoparticles is well defined in this study. The larger particles that were greater than 500 nm, which would be the size of bulk TiO_2 and not considered a nanoparticle, did not penetrate the cell membrane and remained outside the cells.

TiO_2 Nanoparticles: Toxicity Testing

To determine if chemicals are toxic, researchers utilize several markers and tests that reveal whether the chemical creates stress that leads to damage in living tissue.[259] In this Shukla study, human epidermal cells exposed to TiO_2 nanoparticles at concentrations of 8 and 80 µg/ml for 48 hours demonstrated a significant reduction in the ability of the skin cells to survive. In addition, toxicity tests demonstrated significant effects, which increased with increasing concentration of nanoparticles. The tests they utilized were:[260]

1. Oxidative Stress Markers (see below)
2. Micronucleus induced (see below)
3. Cytotoxicity after 48 hours (not after 6 or 24 hours)
4. DNA damage
5. ROS production

1. Oxidative Stress Markers
   A. Antioxidants
      Cells that are exposed to oxidative stress utilize antioxidants to neutralize and stop the potential damage. So by measuring the concentrations of antioxidants researchers can determine whether cells are being stressed. Under stress, the concentration of the antioxidants will decrease as they are consumed in the attempt to protect the cell.

In this study, concentrations of the antioxidant glutathione underwent a statistically significant decline, showing that TiO_2 nanoparticles caused oxidative stress in the cells.

B. Peroxides
Oxidative stress can result in the production of peroxides that are very damaging to the cell, its DNA, and can cause cell death.

In this study, the concentration of hydroperoxide underwent a statistically significantly increase, also showing that TiO_2 nanoparticles caused oxidative stress in the cells.

2. Micronucleus Formation Results from DNA Damage
The micronucleus test is utilized by the U.S. National Toxicology Program to determine the potential of a chemical to cause chromosomal damage that can result in cancer and/or adverse reproductive outcomes. Adverse reproductive outcomes are classified as abnormal chromosome count or chromosomal rearrangements in eggs and sperm that result in:[261]
Birth defects
Fetal deaths
Infertility in animals

Normal cell division:
Chromosomes replicate and divide equally between the two
daughter cells.
Micronucleus cell formation:
Chromosomes broken or damaged by chemicals or radiation
may fail to be included in either of the two daughter nuclei.
Chromosomal material not incorporated into a new nucleus forms
its own nucleus, the micronucleus, which is clearly visible
with a microscope.

In this study, there was significant "micronucleus" creation along side the regular cell nucleus, which illustrates that TiO_2 nanoparticles are genotoxic and damage DNA leading to abnormal cell division.[262]

3. Cytotoxicity after 48 Hours Exposure

These researchers, by extending the exposure time to 48 hours, did find that TiO_2 nanoparticles showed toxic changes in the cell. Studies that only use 6 or even 24 hours of exposure will result in the conclusion that TiO_2 nanoparticles are not toxic.

4 - 5. DNA Damage and ROS Production

A chemical is classified as carcinogenic based on whether it has the ability to induce DNA chromosomal damage as most, if not all, cancers are characterized by specific chromosomal changes. The researchers found:

"The data from the present study demonstrated that TiO_2 nanoparticles induce ROS and oxidative stress leading to genotoxicity (DNA damage) in human epidermal cells. This probable primary genotoxicity mechanism may further trigger signal transduction pathways leading to apoptosis (genetically directed cell self-destruction) or cause interferences with normal cellular processes thereby causing cell death."

In Figure 7, the diagram represents the researchers' theory of how TiO_2 nanoparticles lead to human epidermal (skin) cell damage and death.

TiO₂ Nanoparticles Lead to Human Skin Cell Death

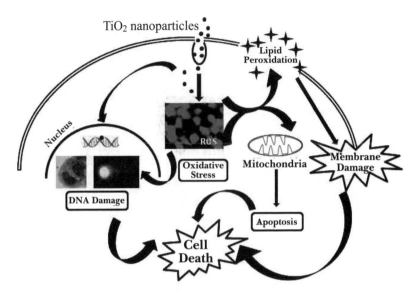

Figure 7. Possible schematic mechanism of TiO₂ nanoparticles induced cellular toxicity in human epidermal cells.

Source: Shukla RK, Sharma V, Pandey AK, Singh S, Sultana S, Dhawan A. ROS-mediated genotoxicity induced by titanium dioxide nanoparticles in human epidermal cells. *Toxicol in Vitro*. 2011. 25(1):231-241. Epub 2010 Nov 17. Reprinted with permission.

The generation of ROS in human skin cells by nanoparticles is shown in Figure 8. Picture A shows the control cells with no nanoparticle exposure, while pictures B through D show a 6 hour exposure to increasing concentrations of TiO₂ nanoparticles at 0.08 µg/ml, 8 µg/ml, and 80 µg/ml, respectively. The amount of fluorescence parallels the amount of ROS that the TiO₂ nanoparticles generate. As the concentration of TiO₂ nanoparticles increases, the greater the number of ROS that are generated, which is shown as increases in the amount of fluorescence that is seen in the pictures.

ROS in Human Skin Cells Generated by TiO₂ Nanoparticles

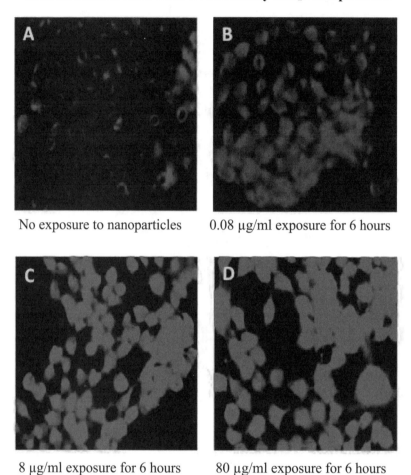

No exposure to nanoparticles   0.08 µg/ml exposure for 6 hours

8 µg/ml exposure for 6 hours   80 µg/ml exposure for 6 hours

Figure 8. Photomicrographs showing the generation of intracellular reactive oxygen species (ROS) using DCFDA dye in human epidermal cells (A) Control cells; (B-D) Cells exposed to TiO₂ NPs (0.08 µg/ml, 8 µg/ml and 80 µg/ml respectively) for 6 hours showing increase in fluorescence (magnification-X200).

Source: Shukla RK, Sharma V, Pandey AK, Singh S, Sultana S, Dhawan A. ROS-mediated genotoxicity induced by titanium dioxide nanoparticles in human epidermal cells. *Toxicol in Vitro.* 2011. 25(1):231-241. Epub 2010 Nov 17. Reprinted with permission.

This study clearly reveals that once TiO_2 nanoparticles are in the body, they have the ability to enter cells where they are then free to cause DNA damage, micronucleus formation, and oxidative stress, which leads to cell death. This raises concern about the safety associated with applications of TiO_2 nanoparticles in consumer products. It is even more imperative to discontinue their use as these researchers also recognized and cited that TiO_2 nanoparticles could gain entry into the body through damaged skin.[262]

TiO_2 Nanoparticles and the Blood-brain Barrier

If the nanoparticles can cross through cell membranes and enter a cell's nucleus, then it makes sense that they can cross the body's protective blood-brain barrier. The body has this barrier in place to protect the brain as it is extremely sensitive and vulnerable to damage by toxic substances. Researchers in a 2010 study published in the *Journal of Nanoscience and Nanotechology* expressed just this concern. They found working with mice and TiO_2 nanoparticles that: "Our results also indicated that TiO_2 nanoparticles might pass through the blood-brain barrier (BBB), and induce the brain injury through oxidative stress response."[263] Indeed, in the 2009 *Toxicology Letters* study discussed earlier, researchers did find TiO_2 nanoparticles in the brain 60 days after being applied to living pigs' ears.[264]

Other researchers, recognizing the possibility that engineered nanoparticles can enter the mammalian body, utilized butyrylcholin-esterase (BChE) (an important enzyme that is present in the brain, blood and nervous system) because it exhibits inhibition when it is exposed to neurotoxins. They found that TiO_2 nanoparticles inhibited BChE in a dose dependent manner, with greater inhibition associated with greater concentrations of the TiO$_2$, which led the researchers to conclude that TiO$_2$ may be neurotoxic.[265]

As studies such as these grow in numbers, there is increasing concern regarding the effects that TiO$_2$ nanoparticles could have on brain function. A study looking directly at brain neurons (nerve cells) exposed to TiO$_2$ nanoparticles found that ROS were generated and the brain neurons died, an effect that also increased in a dose dependent manner with increasing concentrations of the TiO$_2$ nanoparticles.[266]

TiO$_2$ Nanoparticles: Impact on Mammals

2009 *Cancer Research* Study By
UCLA Jonsson Comprehensive Cancer Center

The ubiquitous use of nanosized particles has arisen out of the mistaken idea that since titanium dioxide (TiO$_2$) in bulk form is chemically inert (unreactive), nanosized particles would be also. However, a University of California Los Angeles (UCLA) Jonsson Comprehensive Cancer Center study published in 2009 in *Cancer Reserch* proved that TiO$_2$ acts very differently when it is reduced to nanosized particles. When the researchers exposed mice to TiO$_2$ nanoparticles in their drinking water, they began showing genetic damage by the 5th day.

Compared to regular chemical toxins, their very different chemical reactions resulting from their minute size create a novel mechanism of toxicity. The nanoparticles are so small, the body has no way to eliminate them, so they can go anywhere in the body, accumulating in different organs, including the blood and bone marrow, where they can enter the cell causing oxidative stress, inflammation, and cell death. Being so small, they can also enter the nucleus of the cell, where they increase the risk of cancer, inducing oxidative stress and chromosomal damage, causing breaks in both single and double strand DNA. The study also showed an increase number of "micronucleus" formed that are the result of DNA damage.

TiO$_2$ Nanoparticles in Pregnant Mice: Large DNA Deletions in Their Offspring

This study found that exposing pregnant mice to TiO$_2$ nanoparticles led to a significantly high number of large deletions of DNA in the offspring. Because embryonic cells go through such high turnover during fetal development, they are especially susceptible to this type of oxidative DNA damage.

One of the authors of this study, Dr. Robert Schiestl, UCLA professor of pathology, radiation oncology and environmental health sciences stated: "And some people could be more sensitive to nanoparticles exposure than others. I believe the toxicity of these nanoparticles has not been studied enough." "Given the growing use of TiO$_2$ nanoparticles, these findings raise concern about potential health hazards associated with TiO$_2$ nanoparticles exposure."[267] "These data suggest that we should be concerned about a potential risk of cancer or genetic disorders especially for people exposed to high concentrations TiO$_2$ nanoparticles and that it might be prudent to limit ingestion of TiO$_2$ nanoparticles through nonessential drug additives, food colors, etc." Their results reveal that the TiO$_2$ nanoparticles now being used in most cosmetics pose significant potential for harm to the human fetus.[268] Given this possibility, it behooves us to stop using products with nanoparticles until there is firm confirmation that babies will not be harmed during their critically sensitive neurodevelopment while inside the uterus.

The authors also expressed concern over nanoparticles in spray-on sunscreens as they can be inhaled, because other studies have shown nanoparticles create cancerous tumors in the lungs of mice.[269] Other researchers have confirmed the potential for damage from breathing the nanoparticles. In their review of the literature, looking at the lung being the source of nanoparticle entry, they determined nanoparticles enter the interstitial air spaces in the lungs and are quickly taken up by the tiny air sac alveolar cells and lead to pulmonary toxicity. The exposure of these cells to nanoparticles results in oxidative stress, DNA damage and inflammation leading to the development of fibrous tissue in the lungs. These are unhealthy changes that can result in a condition that is common in coal miners, called pneumoconiosis, which is a chronic respiratory disease caused by inhaling metallic or mineral particles.[270]

TiO_2 Nanoparticles: Create Lung Injury in Mice

In a 2006 study published in *FASEB* (Federation of American Societies for Experimental Biology), researchers found that mice that inhaled a single dose of TiO_2 nanoparticles underwent induced pulmonary toxicity, as demonstrated by pulmonary emphysema, white blood cell accumulation, and epithelial cell death. They also discovered that TiO_2 nanoparticles changed hundreds of gene activating pathways that are involved in cell cycle, cell death, immune system response, and protein activation, one of which is increasing the activity of placenta growth factor (PlGF). The investigators concluded that their results indicate that nanoparticles can induce an inflammatory response that may by caused by PlGF and result in severe pulmonary emphysema.[271]

Chapter 14
Nanoparticle – Impact on Oceans

What Is the Impact on the Oceans
Of the Newer Physical UVA Blockers?

Phytoplankton Decreasing around the World

Phytoplankton are freely floating minute plant organisms that drift with water currents. They consist of diatoms, green algae, cyanobacteria, and dinoflagellates. In fresh water, the green algae colors lakes and ponds, and cyanobacteria can alter the taste of drinking water. In the oceans, phytoplankton is the primary food source of all sea organisms since phytoplankton are eaten by zooplankton, which are prey for small fish and other animals, ultimately supporting the food chain of all marine life. Their abundance in the water varies according to the season, as well as with the light, temperature, and minerals present in the water. As plants, phytoplankton are just like land vegetation as they use carbon dioxide, while giving off oxygen, and converting minerals into a usable form for aquatic and sea animals.

Phytoplankton are not only the critical beginning of the marine food chain, estimates are that they are responsible for producing somewhere between 50–90% of the oxygen in the world. The researchers have calculated that since 1950 there has been a 40% decline of phytoplankton in the world's oceans. The decline has been seen everywhere, except in the Indian Ocean, and in coastal zones where fertilizer run-off from agricultural land has increased nutrient supplies and therefore has supported their growth.[272]

ZnO Nanoparticles: Kill Phytoplankton

Zinc is a necessary and essential micronutrient that is required by over 100 enzymes in the body in order for them to function, however, when the concentration becomes too high due to excessive exposure by ingestion or inhalation, zinc can be toxic to living organisms.[273]

A study published in 2010 in *Environmental Toxicology and Chemistry* showed that ZnO nanoparticles are toxic to the single phytoplankton species of diatom, *Thalassiosira pseudonana*.[274] In another 2010 study in *Environmental Science & Technology*, researchers investigated ZnO nanoparticles impact on population growth rates of four different species of marine phytoplankton that represent three major coastal groups: diatoms; chlorophytes; and prymnesiophytes (photosynthetic algae). They found that ZnO nanoparticles were toxic to the phytoplankton, significantly depressing the growth rate of all four species.[275]

Phytoplankton exposed to ZnO nanoparticles demonstrate significantly depressed growth rates.

One aspect of ZnO nanoparticles is that they are very unstable. They aggregate rapidly in seawater and form into particles greater than 400 nm within 30 minutes. The researchers state that it is difficult to sort out the affects of the nanoparticles from those of free zinc ions, but theorize the nanoparticle toxicity they are seeing is due to the eventual increase of free zinc ions. The researchers concluded that their results suggest the affects on marine organisms by metal oxide nanoparticles will vary with the particle type and organism that is being exposed to them. This study reported that TiO_2 nanoparticles, as compared to ZnO nanoparticles, did not have any measurable effects on growth rates of the phytoplankton.[276]

In a study published in 2010 in *Analytical and Bioanalytical Chemistry*, researchers investigating the potential toxicities of ZnO, either in bulk or nanoparticle form, looked at five different types of marine organisms, which included marine diatoms, the most common algae (phytoplankton), crustaceans, and fish. They found ZnO nanoparticles to be more toxic towards algae, while bulk size ZnO was more toxic to crustaceans. They determined that toxicity was dependent on the organism and on the concentration. Seeing that the nanoparticle instability causes them to form larger aggregates [clumping together] in seawater than the bulk ZnO, which dissolve more readily in seawater, these researchers came to the similar conclusion as those stated above that the nanoparticle toxicity could be due to dissolved Zn ions.[277]

Tio₂ and ZnO Rated Toxic and Harmful to Marine Life

In a study in *Toxicology* also published in 2010, researchers exposed groups that represented the oceans' main food-chain levels: bacteria; algae; crustaceans (daphnids); ciliates; fish; yeasts and nematodes to a variety of nanoparticles that included TiO₂ and ZnO. They found that the algae and crustaceans were the most sensitive of the organisms to the nanoparticles. Ranking them in order of toxicity, they classified ZnO nanoparticles "extremely toxic" and TiO₂ nanoparticles "harmful".[278]

Ecosystem Toxicity

Investigators, looking at the possibility of the nanoparticles being transferred up the food chain to larger and larger organisms, examined mussels and oysters and found significant nanoparticle ingestion of the larger aggregates. They concluded that nanoparticles could have toxicological effects and that they could be transferred up the food chain in the ocean to larger and larger fish, which means they can find their way into our own food supply.[279] Researchers at Rice University in Houston, Texas ended their research study after identifying the toxic effects of both TiO₂ and ZnO nanoparticles with this warning: "The results of this study highlight the need for safe disposal protocols for each of these compounds. Their release into surface or ground waters could have detrimental effects to ecosystem health."[280]

Both UVA and UVB Filters Inflict Harm

There are several variables that are impacting the health of the world's oceans. However, these studies clearly show that both types of sunscreens, the chemical UVB filters and the physical TiO_2 and ZnO nanoparticles used to filter UVA harm marine life. With results this clear cut showing that both types of UV filters contribute to reproductive toxicity and death of aquatic and marine life, it makes no sense to allow the continued use of these products. UVA nanoparticle sunscreens are now at the same place where UVB filters were 30 years ago when they were first incorporated into sunscreen products. There was research published at that time that indicated they had the potential for causing harm, yet those studies were not heeded. As a consequence of disregarding that sunscreen chemicals may be harmful to the body, and approving UVB and UVA chemicals for human use, they are now ubiquitous in our bodies, as well as widely distributed throughout the environment.[281] The use of sunscreens needs to be banned immediately, before more coral and plankton die. These articles demonstrate that TiO_2 nanoparticles are not the safe products we need to use to protect us from skin cancers; rather they create skin cancers, which helps explain why skin cancers and melanomas have increased since the use of sunscreens has been so well embraced by millions of people around the world.

This is also another case of the law of unintended consequences. Nanoparticles are so small, there is no assurance that they will not cross into and migrate through the body, entering cells and the nucleus of the cells, where they have the potential to inflict great harm. Nanoparticles need to be investigated more thoroughly before allowing their continued use. If they go through cell membranes, they can go through the placenta allowing them to enter the cells of the unborn fetus, and since we know they cause DNA damage, nanoparticles could impact our future generations in ways that are only beginning to be recognized.

Part 4 – Sunning Safely

Chapter 15
Infrared Radiation – The Forgotten Wavelengths

The whole promotion of encouraging people to use sunscreens to protect their skin from both skin cancers and photoaging has been accompanied by products that at first only filtered the UVB radiation. The campaign has been tremendously successful as it not only utilized fear of cancer as a motive to induce action, but also pulled on the human obsession with a youthful appearance.[282] However, more and more skin cancers have developed.

Even though manufactures did originally focus their efforts on protecting against UVB, when they realized that UVA radiation was far more implicated in creating cancerous changes than the UVB rays, they expanded their products to include UVA filtering also. Yet, even with the widespread use of these new UVB and UVA filtering sunscreens, termed "broadband sunscreens", there still has been a steady increase in the incidence of skin cancers world-wide.

Now studies are revealing that protection against UVB and UVA is not enough and researchers are beginning to look at the harmful effects of infrared radiation (IR). Throughout the entire time of the mass marketing of sunscreens, there has been no public awareness campaign regarding the fact that IR radiation can create the same type of damage as the UV radiation sunscreens were designed to prevent. The result has been that the public has extended their time in the sun since they no longer have their natural early warning system available — the sunburn — and have been assured they are protected. Since sunscreens have not been designed to also filter out IR radiation, this has been leaving people subject to greater sun exposure than their skin was designed to tolerate without damage. It is important to include in this book how IR affects the skin because existing UV sunscreens do not include protection from this portion of the solar spectrum.

Infrared Rays

The same as UV radiation is broken into subdivisions of UVB and UVA, which correspond to the difference in their ability to penetrate through the different levels of the skin, the IR subdivisions of IRA, IRB, and IRC also happen to correspond with the difference in their ability to penetrate into different levels of the skin.[283] The IRC band is almost completely absorbed by the epidermis. The bands that need to be addressed are the IRA and IRB, as they go through not only the epidermis and the dermis, they penetrate deeper than UV rays by going into the hypodermis layer, also known as the subcutis. Approximately two thirds of the IRB is absorbed by the epidermis, 20% goes into the dermis and 8% passes through to the hypodermis. Of the IRA, 48% infiltrates down into the dermis, while 17% penetrate deep into the hypodermis.[284] See figure 9.

Skin Penetration by IR Solar Rays

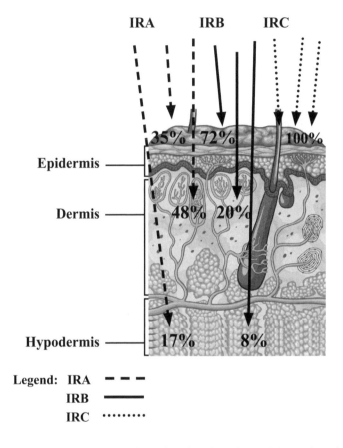

Figure 9. Skin penetration of epidermis, dermis, and hypodermis by IRA, IRB, and IRC radiation.

IR and Skin Cancer

The information above regarding the penetration of the various IR bands of radiation to these deep levels was published in 1931 as part of an article titled "The Penetration of Light through the Skin" in the *American*

Journal of Dermatology. During the years that sunscreens were being formulated and beginning to be promoted, there was evidence published that IR could be harmful. As early as 1978, a researcher called attention to the fact that IR radiation could lead to cancer.[285]

The studies published on IR over the years reveal contradictory findings, which researchers, themselves, state could be the consequence of flaws in the study designs. This has resulted in researchers highlighting the need for more appropriate experiments.[286] Even though there are conflicting findings about the role of IR in the skin, there are several areas where there is no dispute. One thing researchers agree on is that IR radiation produces heat in the skin. The heat generation in the skin is one reason the sun feels good to people, as long as it is not too hot.

In a 1982 *Archives of Dermatological Research* article, a researcher looked at the evidence from the past that heat from cooking fires was found to create skin cancers wherever the heat was most intense on the skin, and determined that heat induces changes in the skin that result in cancer formation. Over 25 years ago, he concluded his findings with warnings that IR radiation had the ability to cause skin cancer. Exposing guinea pigs to either UV or IR or combined UV and IR for 45 weeks, he found that either UV or IR alone caused changes to elastic fibers, changes that were much greater when UV and IR were combined. He stated that because IR radiation makes up approximately 40% of the radiation reaching the earth, the danger connected to IR radiation needed to addressed, and stated physicians can expect to see more patients with IR damage.[287]

Researchers in a 1988 article published in *Seminars in Oncology* stated: "That UVB radiation may play a role in melanoma is supported; at the same time, one cannot exclude the possibility that the action spectrum for melanoma is, instead, the UVA, the visible, or even the NIR (near infrared or IRA) portion of the sunlight spectrum."[288]

Yet, still so little research had been done, that 15 years later a study concluded that the consequences in the cell resulting from IR exposure are virtually unknown.[289] Further, a study published in 2010 states that existing UV protective measures are still ignoring the problems IR radiation can cause.[290]

IR Causes: Photoaging

In 1987, research was published that the full solar spectrum, including IR, has the ability to create photodamage to the skin that would result in its aging.[291] Today, researchers experimenting with infrared (IR) radiation on human buttock skin for 3 times a week for 4 weeks identified connective tissue damage leading them to conclude: "Thus, we suggest that repeated exposure to IR irradiation might induce premature skin aging (photoaging) in human skin in vivo (living)."[292]

One group of researchers concluded that IR plays an important role in the development of photoaging after determining that IR alone, without UV, induces skin wrinkling and thickening. In addition, it increases any wrinkle formation that is induced by UV radiation.[293]

IR Heat Causes Skin Aging

Studies are revealing that IR has many effects that lead to aging of the skin. Heat alone has an effect as the IR absorbed from sunlight raises the temperature of human skin to 104°F (40°C). This IR heat generates ROS, which create DNA damage.[294]

IR Creates ROS in Mitochondria

The IRA radiation generates ROS in the mitochondria, which results in a significant contribution to skin aging.[295] Mitochondria are the energy plants that are located within the cells that provide the essential energy that is required for the cells to do their work.

Currently, this is an area that deserves much investigation to determine what role this plays and what happens when the mitochondria are exposed to IR radiation. It is also important since the mitochondria are essential for the energy of the entire body and responsible for the body's level of metabolism. Since thyroid hormones working at the level of the mitochondria are critical for maintaining a normal thyroid state, interference by IR with mitochondrial function by ROS could be a link to the many thyroid conditions seen today.

IR Damages Collagen and Elastin

As discussed in Chapter 4, collagen and elastin are necessary in our skin to keep it young looking. Research has now uncovered that IR as well as UV decrease collagen and elastin through several pathways, and the decreases they each create result in aging of the skin from both types of radiation.[296]

The combination of high doses of UV, IR and the heat that IR generates makes the blood bring in white blood cells to fill the exposed area for repair. However, white blood cells have enzymes that breakdown the collagen and the elastic fibers that are in the skin, which leads to photoaging.[297]   The use of sunscreens and encouraging people to remain in the sun for longer periods of time results in this type of aging.

IR Protection

Due to the nature of the IR radiation, there are no chemical or physical filters that can be utilized against the IR rays like those that have been developed to filter UVA and UVB radiation. As a result, researchers are looking at ways to stop the effect of IR with chemicals that would work on blocking the impact of radiation on internal cellular mechanisms.

Even though there is preliminary work showing that IR and UVB interact, with IR having a beneficial effect to prevent UVB cell death, some researchers are investigating an agent called mitoquinone (MitoQ), which is a derivative of coenzyme Q10 (CoQ10), that would work on preventing IR radiation from producing ROS in the mitochondria.   Preliminary studies are indicating that it does.[298] MitoQ has been researched as a possible help for Parkinson's disease, due to the observation that there is oxidative stress in mitochondria associated with Parkinson's disease. The latest findings, though, are that it has not proven to be helpful with Parkinson's.[299]

It is important to remember that any chemical they find and want to add to sunscreens needs long-term trials that prove it is safe before it is formulated into products that are released to the public for wide-spread use. So far, research into preventing IR effects in the cells is so new there has not been the time that is necessary to perform the extensive studies that are needed to prove their safety. All chemicals must be examined for generational transmission, as well as for body-wide affects, or we will end up years down the road with millions of people impacted, along with our ecosystem, just as we have been with UVB and UVA filters. Due to their having been released prior to the completion of many studies covered in this book that clearly show their harm, UV sunscreens have caused world-wide damage — damage that may be irreversible to our bodies, our oceans, waterways, and ecosystems.

IR Warnings

Even though this field is still in its infancy, and many studies reveal contradictory findings, several studies from various researchers now conclude that IR can lead to skin aging and that sunscreen formulas need to defend against IR, especially IRA, as well as UVB, and UVA. They also state that at this time there is no current knowledge of whether there are additional wavelengths investigators are not aware of yet that could also contribute to skin damage too.[300] It is important to note researchers warn that; "Skin exposure to infrared (IR) radiation should be limited in terms of irradiance (power), exposure time and frequency in order to avoid acute or chronic damage."[301]

The affects that IR has on human skin have until now largely been ignored. Researchers are saying the new findings about the harm they can cause raise important clinical questions regarding not only photoprotection from the sun, but also surrounding the wide-spread use of IR for skin therapy. There are several groups of researchers who are voicing warnings that unnecessary exposure to IRA radiation from artificial irradiation devices should be avoided.[302]

It is amazing that for over a quarter of a century the public has been assured that all they have to do is slather on UVB filtering sunscreens, and then years later adding UVA filters, with the same assurance they protect from either skin aging or cancer when there was available evidence to the contrary. The studies throughout this book reveal that initially sunscreens did not include protection from the cancer inducing UVA waves and now currently have not included protection from the photoaging and cancer inducing IR radiation. It is no surprise that skin cancers have been on the rise ever since the world-wide campaign of advising everyone to just slather on the sunscreen and you can stay in the sun 5, 15, 20, 30, even 50 times longer than normal, as long as you have a sunscreen on your skin. Yet, as of July 2011, the vast majority of sunscreen products on the market still only protect against UV radiation and do not include coverage of the IR part of the spectrum, which as this chapter conveys results in the same type of damage as UV, especially when staying in the sun way beyond what the skin can naturally tolerate.

IR and Antioxidants

Due to the difficulties in finding effective chemical methods to stop the IR damage or reversing it, it is good to know that applying antioxidants to the skin can protect against detrimental changes that can be caused by IR radiation.[303] Research is proving that antioxidants, especially ones that can target the mitochondria do provide protection against IRA damage. Included among those that have been tested are vitamin C, flavonoids, soy's isoflavone genistein, and the amino acid N-acetylcysteine.[304] Chapter 16 discusses in more detail the antioxidants that have the ability to protect not only from IR, but from the UV rays as well.

Chapter 16
Vitamin D – The Sunshine Vitamin

Vitamin D Metabolism

Vitamin D is a generic term covering various forms that include vitamin D_2 and vitamin D_3.[305] Human skin exposed to sunlight is the vitamin D manufacturing plant for the body. A precursor to vitamin D that is formed from cholesterol, provitamin D, sits in the skin waiting for the UVB radiation range of sunlight to transform it into vitamin D_3, a process that takes place over approximately an 8 hour period.

Vitamin D_3 is the form of the vitamin that is created in the skin in response to UVB light. It is the major circulating form of vitamin D and is considered the most biologically active, therefore it is the best indicator of adequate vitamin D status.

Vitamin D_3 is also identified as 25-hydroxyvitamin D, or with the scientific notation 25(OH)D. Therefore, when a blood test is ordered, one way it can be written on laboratory request slips and reports is 25(OH)D. The laboratory can also test for just vitamin D_3 or vitamin D_2, or total, which would be a measure of both D_3 and D_2 and in the blood. You would then see on the lab request: 25-OHD3; 25- OHD2; or vitamin D, 25-OH, total, respectively.[306]

D_3 is also called cholecalciferol. This term is being included in this book as medical prescriptions today are for the D_2 form of the vitamin, which is termed ergocalciferol. Which vitamin D (D_2 or D_3) people take as a supplement becomes an important point due to studies that compare the efficacy of the two forms of the vitamin. Researchers at the Creighton University Osteoporosis Research Center looking at supplementation of equal amounts of D_2 compared to D_3 (50,000 IU a week for 12 weeks) identified that D_3 is over 80% more effective in its contribution to blood levels, and results in a greater storage of vitamin D in the body than D_2. They concluded: "Given its greater potency and lower cost, D_3 should be the preferred treatment option when correcting vitamin D deficiency."[307]

World-wide Vitamin D Deficiency

Since sunshine is essential for the body to manufacture vitamin D, the world-wide response of using sunscreens to protect against skin cancers and skin aging has led to a resurgence of vitamin D deficiency in many countries. The following articles are clarion calls that highlight the depth and breadth of this arising epidemic.

The UK Telegraph Headline – Friday 10 September 2010

Vitamin D Health Warning for the Children Who Shun the Sun

"Paranoia about sun exposure and indoor lifestyles are causing life-threatening health problems for children due to vitamin D deficiency, a new study claims.

Casualty departments are dealing with dozens of emergency cases where infants are having seizures as a direct result of not getting enough vitamin D, which is essential for healthy teeth and bones.

In one case, a baby suffered brain damage after a fit.

The study said the extreme cases are part of an escalating problem of a deficiency of the vitamin, which the body makes when exposed to sunlight.

The report in the *London Journal of Primary Care* blames indoor lifestyles and the use of high sun protection factor creams for a health issue unheard of a decade ago.

The findings have prompted experts to call for vitamin D pills to be made more widely available on the NHS (National Health Service, UK), especially for pregnant women."[308]

The UK Telegraph headline – Friday 28 January 2011

Middle Class Children Suffering Rickets

Professor Nicholas Clarke, consultant orthopedic surgeon at Southampton General Hospital and professor of pediatric orthopedic surgery at the University of Southampton, warned that parents covering children in sunscreen and limiting their time outside in the sunshine has led to the reemergence of rickets in English middle class children.

Identifying that over 20% of children have significant bone problems due to low vitamin D, Dr. Clarke stated: "In my 22 years at Southampton General Hospital, this is a completely new occurrence in the south that has evolved over the last 12 to 24 months and we are seeing cases across the board, from areas of deprivation up to the middle classes, so there is a real need to get national attention focused on the dangers this presents."

"This is almost certainly a combination of the modern lifestyle, which involves a lack of exposure to sunlight, but also covering up in sunshine, and we're seeing cases that are very reminiscent of 17th century England."

Dr. Clarke added: "We are facing the daunting prospect of an area like Southampton, where it is high income, middle class and leafy in its surroundings, seeing increasing numbers of children with rickets, which would have been inconceivable only a year or so ago."[309]

Vitamin D's Role in Body-wide Health
Reemergence of Rickets

Rickets is a disease that was so rampant in 17th century England due to the city children not having enough sunlight, it was dubbed the "17th century disease". Rickets continued to be common in the late 1800s and into the early 1900s. Without sufficient vitamin D, minerals required for making strong bones are not absorbed from the intestinal tract so the bones become soft and deformed. When this happens in infants and children the condition is termed rickets, in adults it is called osteomalacia, or adult rickets. It shows up in children as bow legged or knock kneed deformities, in adults it is experienced as muscle weakness, and bone pain or fractures.[310]

Rickets virtually disappeared with recognition of the importance of sunlight and with vitamin D fortification of foods. However, newspaper articles like the ones above highlight that rickets has re-emerged in the United Kingdom, and has returned in the U.S. as well.[311]

In a study conducted in 2005, English researchers cautioned that low vitamin D status was a prevalent health problem when they determined that approximately 20% of the population had what they consider deficient levels at less than 25 ng/mL (62.5 nmol/L) vitamin D in their blood. Seeing that there was a significant decline in men from 1995 vitamin D levels, they concluded there was an urgent need for a uniform policy on assessment and dietary supplementation of vitamin D in older people.[312]

Due to high latitude sun not being strong enough for vitamin D production in the skin during the winter, countries in high latitudes such as the United Kingdom (latitude 51° N) are the ones that are demonstrating the high percentage of extreme overt symptoms the newspaper articles above were discussing, like bone deformities and seizures that can occur as a result of low vitamin D levels throughout pregnancy and in the first few months of life.

However, the lower latitude countries where there is still enough radiation from the sun during winter for some vitamin D synthesis, the harmful effects that minimal vitamin D blood levels can create do not show up as dramatically, and are therefore more difficult to identify. Vitamin D is involved in so many aspects of the healthy normal functioning of the body, the diminishing levels that occur due to liberal sunscreen application, or hiding from the sun, can result in many conditions that are not being directly linked to the overall decreasing vitamin D levels found in the population. Yet, identifying lower than healthful vitamin D levels is critical for the promotion of everyone's general body-wide health.

In 2008 looking at the statistics of vitamin D status world-wide, two researchers concluded:

"Vitamin D deficiency is now recognized as a pandemic. The major cause of vitamin D deficiency is the lack of appreciation that sun exposure in moderation is the major source of vitamin D for most humans. Very few foods naturally contain vitamin D, and foods that are fortified with vitamin D are often inadequate to satisfy either a child's or an adult's vitamin D requirement."[313]

Another researcher also in 2008 emphasized that action is urgently needed in tackling the global burden of rickets and osteomalacia.[314] In a January 2011 article, the continued problem led other researchers to plead for urgent action citing the re-emergence of rickets and the public health burden of low vitamin D status as being already apparent.[315]

Decreased Solar Radiation = Decreased Vitamin D = Increased Cancer

A 2009 *Annals of Epidemiology* analysis of the studies that have been published in relation to cancer and the amount of solar radiation and vitamin D levels has provided evidence that is ". . . scientifically strong enough to warrant use of vitamin D in cancer prevention, and as a component of treatment."[316]

Many of the conditions and diseases that are appearing to be associated with vitamin D deficiencies are more prevalent in the higher latitudes, which would reflect that people living at the high latitudes and do not experience as much solar radiation in the winter have correspondingly lower vitamin D levels. Indeed, studies show that people living in higher latitudes have more cancers and more deaths from the types of cancers that appear to be influenced by vitamin D, which include pancreas, prostate, ovarian, uterine (endometrial), breast, bladder, and colon cancers.[317]

Croatia is at the higher latitude of 45° N. As stated earlier almost 70% of the population state they use sunscreens, and in addition to increasing skin cancer and melanoma rates, hormone-dependent cancer incidence is also on the rise, particularly in the younger age group of less than 35 years old. From 1994 to 2005, breast cancer incidence rates increased by 21%, rising from 55.6 per 100,000 to 67.4 per 100,000. Testicular cancer increase was even greater as its incidence rates increased from 3.4 per 100,000 in 1994 to 12.8 per 100,000 in 2005. The researchers stated the increase in the younger population may be due to a complex mixture that includes environmental estrogen exposure.[318]

Sunshine may be of benefit even for melanoma. A study on U.S. Navy personal shows that those who worked inside had a higher incidence rate of melanoma, compared with those who worked both inside and outside. This finding combined with the fact that more melanoma was found on the trunk of the body, which was protected from the sun, compared to the sun exposed areas of the head and arms, led the researchers to theorize that the sun has a protective effect when the skin has brief, regular exposure.[319] As with everything, moderation is generally okay, but excess is harmful.

Why Vitamin D Is Important to General Health

Even though it is termed a vitamin, the structure and mode of action of vitamin D is similar to the hormones that are classified as steroid hormones. All steroid hormones are made from the parent structure, cholesterol. The most commonly known ones are testosterone, estradiol, progesterone, and cortisol.[320]

How and where the cholesterol originates that eventually becomes vitamin D within the skin is currently part of intense investigation, without all questions being answered.[321] However, since vitamin D is formed from cholesterol, taking cholesterol lowering drugs (i.e., statin drugs) can influence the amount of vitamin D the body can manufacture. New studies as to whether the level of vitamin D is lowered or raised when taking statins are reporting conflicting results at this point. However, it is wise for anyone taking cholesterol lowering drugs to keep in mind that all the hormones that are made from cholesterol (e.g., estrogens, progesterone, testosterone, and vitamin D) are impacted while on medications that disrupt the formation of cholesterol in the body. As all of these steroid hormones are critical for health, it is important to make sure you keep your cholesterol levels high enough so the body can manufacture the levels of hormones that are necessary for maintaining good health.

Vitamin D plays a central role in muscle functioning. Studies are beginning to show that individuals taking statin drugs who start to have problems with weakened muscle function (i.e., statin-induced myalgia) have low vitamin D blood levels, which could be contributing to this potentially debilitating and possibly even life-threatening condition.[322]

In the body, hormones work in the tissues and organs whose cells have receptors that are specific for the particular hormone. Once attached to the receptor, the hormones become available to perform their functions that are necessary for the health of the specific system.

Vitamin D's impact throughout almost every system in the body is proven by the fact that vitamin D receptors are found not just in the skin, but also in the brain, heart, ovaries, testicles, prostate, breast, small intestine, colon, bone forming cells, white blood cells, as well as in the cells of the pancreas. This shows that vitamin D is essential for all these organs to function as they should.[323]

Vitamin D Deficiency Can Result In:
Bone loss
    Children:[324]
        Growth retardation, bone deformities, rickets
    Adults:[325]
        Osteopenia, osteoporosis, increased falls, increased
        fractures, osteomalacia

In addition to bone loss, vitamin D deficiency is associated with:[326]
    Increase in all cancers[327]
    Autoimmune diseases:[328]
        Hashimoto's disease
        Autoimmune thyroid disease (thyroid antibodies)
    Hypertension (high blood pressure)[329]
    Cardiovascular disease[330]
    Strokes[331]
    Increased infections:[332]
        Vaginal infections[333]
    Decreased muscle function:[334]
        Urinary incontinence
        Women's pelvic floor disorders[335]
    Musculoskeletal pain, persistent and nonspecific (e.g.,
        fibromyalgia, CFS)[336]

Increased cesarean section deliveries[337]
Depression:[338]
    Seasonal Adjustment Disorder (SAD) in winter[339]
Metabolic syndrome[340]
Obesity[341]
Type 2 diabetes mellitus (vitamin D is involved in glucose metabolism)[342]
Inflammatory bowel disease (adults and children)[343]
Crohn's disease[344]
Psoriasis[345]
Cognitive impairment in elderly (diet less than 35 mcg/week)[346]
Low vitamin D during pregnancy:
    Newborn multiple sclerosis (MS)[347]
    Schizophrenia[348]
    Type 1 diabetes mellitus[349]

The diagram in Figure 10 was utilized in a *Workshop on Vitamin D* that was presented by the University of California, Riverside. It highlights all the systems throughout the body that require vitamin D and clearly demonstrates how decreases in this sunshine vitamin impact the health of the entire body.

Organs Impacted and Diseases Associated with Low Vitamin D

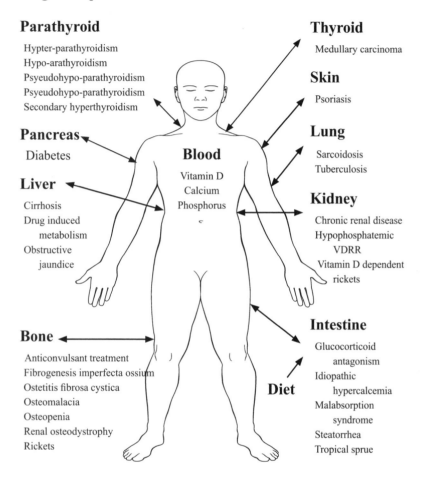

Parathyroid

Hypter-parathyroidism
Hypo-arathyroidism
Psyeudohypo-parathyroidism
Psyeudohypo-parathyroidism
Secondary hyperthyroidism

Pancreas

Diabetes

Liver

Cirrhosis
Drug induced
  metabolism
Obstructive
  jaundice

Blood

Vitamin D
Calcium
Phosphorus

Bone

Anticonvulsant treatment
Fibrogenesis imperfecta ossium
Ostetitis fibrosa cystica
Osteomalacia
Osteopenia
Renal osteodystrophy
Rickets

Thyroid

Medullary carcinoma

Skin

Psoriasis

Lung

Sarcoidosis
Tuberculosis

Kidney

Chronic renal disease
Hypophosphatemic
VDRR
Vitamin D dependent
  rickets

Intestine

Glucocorticoid
  antagonism
Idiopathic
  hypercalcemia
Malabsorption
  syndrome
Steatorrhea
Tropical sprue

Diet

Figure 10. Organs affected along with diseases and conditions that arise from vitamin D deficiency.

Source: University of California Riverside Website. Norman AW. Disease and Vitamin D. Available at: http://vitamind.ucr.edu/disease. html. Accessed February 2, 2011. Reprinted with permission.

Another whole book would be required to describe the biochemistry of why inadequate levels of vitamin D can lead to all the disease states listed. Why bone loss occurs is an illustration of the domino effects that happen when vitamin D is not at optimum levels.

Why Vitamin D Deficiency Results in Bone Loss

Vitamin D affects start with absorption of nutrients from food. The rickets in children and osteoporosis in adults discussed earlier are the result of low vitamin D, because when levels are too low, only 10–15% of calcium and 60% of phosphorus is absorbed from the food we eat, and since bones need these minerals in their structure, strong bones cannot be built.[350]

The decreased absorption of calcium through the intestines compounds the problems, as calcium levels in the blood can decrease so low that the body starts pulling calcium out of the bones that are already formed in order to maintain the many calcium dependent cellular functions that are essential for the preservation of life.[351]

Since bones require both calcium and phosphorus for adequate mineralization to build and maintain their strength, the low vitamin D levels result in the weakened bone structure such as that seen with rickets, osteomalacia, and osteoporosis.

Laboratory Testing

Laboratory tests are available to determine an individual's vitamin D level. Today, with the greater awareness of rampant vitamin D deficiency, more physicians are adding vitamin D to the blood testing that is performed in routine physicals. Keep in mind, however, that blood tests only provide a snap shot of that particular day's level in the blood.

Throughout this book both the English and the metric, also known as the International System (SI) of measurements, are included with the English listed first followed by the SI measurement. For vitamin D blood levels, these are ng/mL (English) and nmol/L (metric SI).

Laboratory Testing is Only an Estimation

Laboratory values are really only a ball park figure and just an estimation of the true value due to what laboratorians call an inherent problem with many laboratory tests: "measurement uncertainty". A study comparing 4 different vitamin D laboratory assays that are in use today on the same sample in triplicate over a 5 day period found a variation of 20%, 16%, and 11% for vitamin D average content of 14 ng/mL (35 nmol/L), 32 ng/mL (80 nmol/L), and 50 ng/mL (126 nmol/L), respectively. This means that a lab value of 14 ng/mL (35 nmol/L) could actually be anywhere between 11–17 ng/mL (28–42 nmol/L). If the value is near 32 ng/mL (80 nmol/L), it could actually be somewhere between 27–37 ng/mL (67–93 nmol/L). If the value is 50 ng/mL (126 nmol/L), it can range between 45–56 ng/mL (112–140 nmol/L).[352]

This is true for many laboratory tests and illustrates that laboratory reports should only be used as guidelines for monitoring your vitamin D status. There is a more reliable testing methodology (liquid chromatography-tandem mass spectrometry), but not all laboratories utilize it. Considering how important adequate vitamin D levels are it would be best to make sure that your values are higher than your target goal to assure you have sufficient vitamin D for your health.[353]

Vitamin D: Optimal Blood Levels

There is general agreement regarding the levels of vitamin D_3 in the blood that are considered the minimal requirement.

Blood levels of vitamin D 25(OH)D are considered:[354]

	English	SI
Deficient when below	20 ng/mL	50 nmol/L
Insufficient when between	21–29 ng/mL	51–74 nmol/L
Sufficient when greater than	30 ng/mL	75 nmol/L

Experts from around the world looking at the existing literature agree that 20 ng/mL (50 nmol/L) is the lower threshold limit, and values below this cutoff defines a person at risk for rickets and osteomalacia. The levels that are considered healthy and prevent disease are higher, however, there is much disagreement as to what levels are considered to be high enough.

World-wide studies provide a range for recommended sufficient blood levels of vitamin D_3. There is some agreement that the minimum vitamin D_3 blood level is at least 30 ng/mL (75 nmol/L), while several recommend the most beneficial levels would be between 36–44 ng/mL (90–110 nmol/L), yet still others suggest levels from 30 to as high as 80 ng/mL (75–200 nmol/L) would be the most supportive. For children, one researcher recommends 20–60 ng/mL (50–150 nmol/L) would be most optimal.[355]

Sun Exposure Time

An international group of experts determined that seasonal exposure to the sun's UVB radiation was the major contributor to vitamin D_3 levels, while vitamin D_3 from food contributed less.[356] There are no simple guidelines as to how much sunlight a person needs a day to maintain a healthy level of vitamin D in the blood.

Many factors impact the amount of vitamin D_3 that is generated. The amount of radiation from the winter sun at high latitudes on the planet, such as those found in northern Europe, is not enough to generate the formation of vitamin D_3 in the skin. Also, in the summer, it is the mid-day sun that leads to a greater amount of vitamin D_3 formation. Additionally, older people have a dramatic age-related decline in their ability to create vitamin D_3, as their skin manufactures only approximately 25% as much vitamin D when compared to younger skin with the same UV exposure.[357]

Melanin Competes for UVB Radiation

There is competition between the vitamin D_3 precursor and melanin in the skin for the UVB radiation that enters the skin, which limits the amount of vitamin D_3 the body can produce.[358] Since melanin absorbs the UVB radiation that enters the skin, the darker a person's skin, the less UVB radiation waves are available to create vitamin D_3. Studies show that fair or light skin persons generally have adequate levels of vitamin D_3 during the summer and additional supplementation is not necessary at that time. This is not true for those with darker skin, and they do need to supplement all year with vitamin D_3 to attain blood levels that are considered to be protective from all the conditions that can arise from deficient vitamin D_3 levels.[359]

There are conflicting results from studies in regards to the amount of time that is needed to spend in the sun to achieve adequate vitamin D levels in the body. The problem is there are so many variables: much depends on the location on the planet alone; the latitude on the earth; season of the year when the sun exposure takes place; the time of day; the amount of reflection afforded by water or snow; the weather and if there are clouds; all tremendously influence the amount of solar radiation that comes through to the skin. There are also individual differences that greatly influence the amount of radiation that is absorbed, which in turn affects how much of the provitamin D is transformed into vitamin D_3. Much depends on a person's age and the amount of melanin as well as cholesterol in their skin. It becomes difficult for any study to account for all of these variables.[360] Sunshine cannot lead to an overdose of vitamin D_3 as the body has its own built-in, self-regulating brake for when there is too much UVB radiation due to constant or excess exposure to sunlight. When UVB overexposure occurs, the excess sunlight reverses the process and the precursor (provitamin D) and the vitamin D_3 that was created begin to breakdown into other products.[361]

So how much sunlight is enough? There have been many studies conducted to answer this question, and there have been many answers, but because of all the variables involved there is little agreement among them. The remainder of this section will highlight the recommendations from the studies that have been published.

For comparing UVB radiation doses, a scale that utilizes the amount of solar radiation that induces the start of erythema (reddening that is just short of developing a sunburn) of the skin is termed the Minimal Erythemal Dose or MED. Experts measuring exposure to what they determined to be "1 standard MED of UVB exposure" to the sun per week found it increased blood levels of vitamin D_3 by 2.5–5 ng/mL (1–2 nmol/L).[362]

In order to determine the amount of vitamin D that would be generated from a certain amount of time in the sun, researchers in one study used calculations from a computer model that utilized the standard that 1/4 of a MED on 1/4 of the body surface would provide approximately the equivalent of 1,000 IU (400 mcg) of oral vitamin D. From this they calculated that at high noon (time of day of the most solar radiation) April through October, a person with light skin with a quarter of their body exposed who spent 3–8 minutes in the sun at the latitude of Boston, Massachusetts (latitude 42° N), or a person who spent 3–6 minutes any month of the year in Miami, Florida (latitude 25° N) would only synthesize approximately 400 IU (160 mcg) of vitamin D_3.[363]

In 1995, one researcher found that in less than 20 hours of whole-body exposure to simulated solar UVB radiation (equal to 1 standard MED) increased blood levels of vitamin D to a peak of 20 ng/mL (52 nmol/L), and stayed above 16 ng/mL (40 nmol/L) for over 60 hours. Based on this, he recommended that white, elderly people in Boston expose their hands, face, and arms two to three times a week to the amount of time in the sunlight that for them would be below the level of reddening of the skin. For example, if in July they would normally experience a sunburn after 30 minutes exposure to the sun, then exposure of 5–10 minutes would be sufficient to provide adequate vitamin D levels.[364] The Mayo Clinic's Website states that 10 minutes of exposure a day can supply the average person with their body's vitamin D requirements.[365]

In attempts to find a compromise to determine how much sunlight is required to provide healthful levels of vitamin D_3 while protecting the skin from damage, U.K. researchers exposed Caucasians to simulated sunlight exposure of a slightly greater than 1 standard MED dose, while in shorts and T-shirts 3 times a week for 6 weeks. There were 90% who reached the suboptimal level of 20 ng/mL (50 mmol/L), while only approximately 25% were able to achieve a vitamin D_3 blood level that is considered protective at 32 ng/mL (80 mmol/L).[366]

During the winter in the United Kingdom the seasonal variation in circulating vitamin D_3 in Caucasians falls below 25 nmol/L. During the winter and spring, this low level is found in 10% for those residing in south, while over 20% for those living in the higher latitude in the north of England have this low level.[367] High winter vitamin D_3 blood levels are found in the people with the highest summer vitamin D_3 blood levels, which were attained by those who had a preference for staying in the sun instead of the shade during summer, as well as a skin type that allowed for longer sun exposure.[368]

In another study, to determine the amount of drop in vitamin D in winter, researchers drew blood on over 100 men and women in the

U.K. over a 12 month period. Due to summer sun, September blood levels were the highest at 28 ng/mL (70 nmol/L), which dropped to 18 ng/mL (45 nmol/L) in February. For those who attained a summer high between 30–35 ng/mL (75–88 nmol/L), their winter low in February was 20 ng/mL (50 nmol/L).[369]

One set of researchers determined that at the high latitude of the U.K., exposing the skin for short periods to the summer (March to October) mid-day peak intense UVB radiation produces protective levels of vitamin D, with minimal risk of sunburn and cell damage.[370]

Even with this evidence, a researcher warned that attempting to improve vitamin D₃ levels in the blood by sun exposure compromises skin health.[371] However, this same researcher also identified that studies do not show that the use of sunscreen reduces the incidence of melanoma. In a 2009 article published in the *British Journal of Dermatology* he stated:

"The formulation and absorption properties of sunscreens have undoubtedly improved over recent years. Yet the data to support these modern products as an effective means of reducing the incidence of melanoma incidence remains elusive and will do so for at least another decade."

"Despite the lack of evidence demonstrating the efficacy of modern sunscreens in preventing melanoma, it is argued that it would be irresponsible not to encourage their use, along with other sun protection strategies, as a means of combating the year-on-year rise in melanoma incidence."[372]

Yet, if the primary use of sunscreens is to protect from melanoma and the evidence is clearly showing that they do not, how can their continued use still be encouraged, much less justified?

Since there is no benefit from prolonged sun exposure due to the resulting loss of vitamin D, some investigators state that it is possible to balance the need for vitamin D with the goal of avoiding sunburn, which is the main goal in reducing the risk of melanoma.[373]

Dietary Intake of Vitamin D

The Mayo Clinic Website advises:

"If you eat a balanced diet and get outside in the sunshine at least 1-1/2 to 2 hours a week, you should be getting all the vitamin D you need."[374]

With decades of sun shielding behavior, combined with lack of sufficient sun due to the season and/or latitude, more than 50% of the world's population is at risk for vitamin D deficiency. This even includes those who maintain a healthy diet, because the food we eat today does not provide adequate amounts of vitamin D.[375]

The best sources of natural vitamin D_3 are salt water fish like salmon, herring, sardines, along with fish liver oils, dried Shiitake mushrooms, and whole egg yolks. Veal, beef, butter, and vegetable oils provide only small quantities, followed by plants, fruits, and nuts that supply even less. Since there are very few foods that naturally contain vitamin D, it is difficult for natural sources to supply the minimum vitamin D_3 required for either adults or children.[376] The difficulty in achieving sufficient protective blood levels through diet is what led to the artificial fortification of foods containing the fat that is necessary for absorption of the D_3, such as milk, margarine and butter, cereals, and chocolate mixes in countries like the U.S.[377] For most people today, however, the vitamins that our processed foods are fortified with will not reach the levels required to maintain adequate levels of vitamin D.

The dietary requirement for vitamin D supplementation in the winter is dependent on the blood levels that each individual was able to achieve from their summer sun exposure. Vitamin D_3 has a half-life in the body of 2 to 3 weeks. This means that 2 to 3 weeks after exposure there is still 1/2 the amount circulating in the blood that was generated by the sun, an amount that keeps reducing by 1/2 every additional 2 to 3 weeks.[378]

There is some disagreement in the U.S. over whether there is a vitamin D deficiency in the population and whether a deficiency can lead to a multitude of disease states, what blood levels are required to maintain health, and what supplementation dosage would be needed to achieve those blood levels. A report by the U.S. Institute of Medicine brought these disagreements to the forefront in 2011.

U.S. Institute of Medicine 2011 Report On
Dietary Requirements for Calcium and Vitamin D

The U.S. Institute of Medicine (IOM) Committee concluded that scientific evidence does support a cause-and-effect relationship of calcium and vitamin D in skeletal health. However, they felt there was limited, inconclusive and insufficient evidence to determine the nutritional requirements for the other disorders that have been linked to vitamin D deficiency. "The committee concluded that the prevalence of vitamin D inadequacy in North America has been overestimated. Urgent research and clinical priorities were identified, including reassessment of laboratory ranges for 25-hydroxyvitamin D, to avoid problems of both under treatment and over treatment." Their recommendations for vitamin D intake to obtain a blood level of at least 20 ng/mL (50 nmol/L) for maintaining bone health are:[379]

Age	Daily Intake Requirement*
1 to 70	600 IU (15 mcg)
over 70	800 IU (20 mcg)

* The same as blood levels are listed in both English and SI, the amount of vitamin D in foods and supplements is listed in the English, which is International Units (IU), and by the SI metric units, which is micrograms (mcg). For vitamin D3: 40 IU =1 microgram (mcg); 1 IU = 0.025 mcg.

These recommendations, however, are challenged by doctors who have researched and published many studies regarding vitamin D over the years. After hearing reports that physicians were decreasing their vitamin D recommendations to their patients as a result of the 2011 IOM recommendations, researchers who had previously served on the IOM panel during the drafting of their 1997 guidelines for vitamin D and calcium, Drs. Robert Heaney and Michael Holick, responded that they "respectfully dissent" against many of the IOM's findings and recommendations. They stated the evidence demonstrates that only a small fraction of the population has vitamin D levels that are sufficient enough for maintaining a healthy body. Citing the studies that show higher daily intake is important for skeletal health, they proposed that the IOM recommended guidelines should have been worded more appropriately as:

"We do not know whether taking more vitamin D than we are currently recommending will help you, but it could, and we can assure you that supplemental intakes up to at least 4,000 IU per day are safe."

They further went on to state that when it comes to nutrients utilized or produced by the body, as opposed to drugs that are foreign to the body, ". . . which do carry an appropriately heavy requirement for proof," using guidelines requiring for the burden of proof to be on studies to prove higher levels are beneficial is an incorrect approach. Rather daily intake should be based on what the human body has evolved with. Citing there is evidence that indicates humans have had an approximate intake of 4000 IU (100 mcg) a day, or even 2–3 times higher, to produce the blood levels between 40–80 ng/mL (100–200 nmol/L), which Drs. Heaney and Holick have determined are required for maintaining good health.[380]

Their in-depth research of vitamin D has resulted in their conclusion that 400 IU (10 mcg) of vitamin D a day produces barely noticeable changes in blood levels, and is not near enough to increase blood levels up to what is now considered sufficient enough to provide for the body's requirements. Since blood testing has advanced enough that the response to the 400 IU L (10 mcg) can now be measured and is found to only be about 2.8 ng/mL (7.0 nmol/L), these doctors stated this amount would: ". . . fall into a curious zone between irrelevance and inadequacy" in regards to the taking of only 400 IU (10 mcg) a day. The only way this small amount would be sufficient, would be if people also had sun exposure. These doctors state that their research shows even 2,000 IU (50 mcg) per day is still too low, and should be at least double that amount. This is based on their finding that 3,800 IU (95 mcg) per day were needed to sustain a summer blood level of 28 ng/mL (70 nmol/L) in 67 men in Omaha, Nebraska (latitude 41° N) over a 20 week period of the winter.[381]

For pregnant women who have good dietary sources of vitamin D, the currently recommended 400 IU (10 mcg) a day is not a high enough intake. At this level, blood samples show that 73% of women and 80% of their newborn babies are below the deficiency level of 20 ng/mL (50 nmol/L).[382]

Researchers around the world have developed various recommendations for optimal daily intake of vitamin D supplementation. It appears very confusing, but again really depends on the individual and their particular biochemistry, what vitamin D level they start with, what vitamin D blood level is desired, as well as the latitude where they live, and how much they are in the sunshine. As a result the range of suggested dietary intake from supplements varies from 360–5,000 IU (9–125 mcg) a day.[383] The 2008 dietary intake recommendations of the 3rd U.S. National Health and Nutrition Examination Survey suggested:[384]

Starting Blood Levels	Daily Intake Required
Below 22 ng/mL (55 nmol/L)	5000 IU (125 mcg)
Above 22 ng/mL (55 nmol/L)	3800 IU (95 mcg)

An article posted June 15, 2009 on the Web based news source for physicians, *Medscape*, listed the recommendations for healthy blood levels and the daily intake that would be necessary to achieve those levels. They are:[385]

Blood Levels – Desired   Daily Intake Required

35–40 ng/mL (90–100 nmol/L)   800–1,000 IU (20–25 mcg)

Several studies have looked at the differences in vitamin D levels in response to sun exposure of those with Black skin (more melanin) compared to those with White skin. In 2010, investigators at University of California, Davis calculated the difference in dietary daily requirements to achieve basic vitamin D levels in the blood. They are:[386]

White Skin (in winter)

Blood Levels – Desired   Daily Intake Required

30 ng/mL (75 nmol/L)   1,300 IU (32.50 mcg)

Black Skin (all year)

20 ng/mL (50 nmol/L)   2,000 IU (50 mcg)

A 2007 study of postmenopausal African American women determined the requirements to achieve blood levels greater than 30 ng/mL (75 nmol/L) and to maintain adequate vitamin D levels all year. The amount is dependent on the starting blood levels and more is needed if vitamin D levels are below 18 ng/mL (45 nmol/L).[387]

Black Skin (all year)

Starting Blood Level	Blood Level – Desired	Daily Intake Required
Below 18 ng/mL (45 nmol/L)	30 ng/mL (75 nmol/L)	4000 IU (100 mcg)
Above 18 ng/mL (45 nmol/L)	30 ng/mL (75 nmol/L)	2800 IU (70 mcg)

Research in Poland is driven by the fact that their country only has sunlight that is effective enough for skin synthesis of vitamin D from April to September due to their latitude (51° N). They also recognize that sunscreens can reduce the synthesis of vitamin D by 90%, and they are seeing the prevalence of vitamin D insufficiency continually increasing. For these reasons, they state that diet and supplements play important roles to maintain sufficient levels when the sun is less available. They state the general requirements for adults and obese children is between 800–1,000 IU/day (20–25 mcg/day) and should be taken all year for those who do not get adequate sun in the summer. However, when it comes to recommending dosages, they state that the variability of vitamin D amongst individuals requires that monitoring of individual 25(OH)D levels must be considered in order to define the optimal dosage for each person.[388]

Since vitamin D is a fat soluble vitamin, it means that it can accumulate in the fatty tissues of the body. Therefore, the Mayo Clinic recommended the maximum dose should be 2,000 IU (50 mcg) daily, over concern that higher doses may lead to toxicity.[389] However, studies indicate there is no toxicity with higher doses. Indeed, the *Merck Manual* (medical textbook of diagnosis and therapy) states it would take adults several months of taking 50,000 IU/day (1,250 mcg) before it could produce toxicity. For infants it would take 1–4 months at 40,000 IU/day (1,000 mcg) to produce toxicity.[390]

Cholesterol Levels More Important than Melanin?

Even though studies have routinely shown that there is a higher daily intake requirement for individuals with darker pigmentation, there are new studies that indicate the increased melanin in darker pigmented skin may not be the limiting factor for the amount of vitamin D manufactured in the skin in response to sunlight. They reveal that the amount of vitamin D manufactured is more the result of a higher baseline of both vitamin D and total cholesterol, rather than based on amount of skin pigmentation. This research is still ongoing, however, and more will continue to be revealed as to which is the most important factor, or if it is a mixture of factors.[391]

Sunscreens and Vitamin D

Even though some researchers state that sunscreens do not reduce vitamin D levels, other researchers have confirmed they have determined that even small amounts of sunscreen substantially reduces vitamin D_3 levels. In 1987, researchers exposed using human volunteers to one erythema dose of UV radiation after applying a single application of the sunscreen PABA. Their blood levels of vitamin D_3 after exposure remained essentially the same: 5 ng/mL (12.5 nmol/L) on day of application and 4 ng/mL (10 nmol/L) on day 1. This is in contrast to the controls not using PABA, who experienced increases in their blood levels from 1.5 ng/mL up to 25 ng/mL (62.5 nmol/L).[392] Since vitamin D is appearing to be more and more important in preventing diseases, including cancers, in a 2008 article a researcher called for more studies looking into the potential of sunscreens to block vitamin D formation from the sun.[393] This recommendation of reviewing sunscreen's potential for diminishing vitamin D_3 is critical when studies show that a sunscreen with a SPF 8 reduces vitamin D_3 production by more than 92.5%, while a SPF of 15 reduces the production in the skin by more than 99%.[394]

The number of health conditions that are becoming recognized as arising from lack of sufficient amount of vitamin D that has accompanied the public education campaign to shield from the sun has been put into the monetary cost to the American public. One study determined that for the year 2004 just estimating the cancer costs that result from vitamin D insufficiency due to insufficient exposure to solar UVB radiation, combined with inadequate diet and supplements are estimated to be between $40–56 billion. This is in contrast to the estimate for the costs involved for excess UV exposure to be approximately $6–7 billion. The researcher states that the estimate of $40–56 billion is on the low side, as it does not take into consideration the protection vitamin D affords against infectious diseases alone, neither does it take into account the cost of other conditions, such as osteoporosis.[395]

While the additional research is being performed it is essential to understand vitamin D3 and its role in the overall health of the body. Sunscreen use has had consequences with its screening out the vital ultraviolet B radiation that is required by the body for it to manufacture vitamin D3.[396]

Many studies have identified that vitamin D3 deficiency has become recognized as a world-wide epidemic. One researcher stated in an article published in *Advances in Experimental Medicine and Biology*: "There needs to be a renewed appreciation of the beneficial effect of moderate sunlight for providing all humans with their vitamin D requirement for health."[397] The conclusion of one group of researchers is that as long as there is access to sunlight on a regular basis for people living at the latitude of the U.S., sufficient vitamin D3 can be produced with no need for a dietary supplement requirement for this vitamin.[398]

The Health Council of the Netherlands in a governmental report recommended educating the public that spending at least 15 minutes a day outdoors in combination with a healthy diet generates sufficient vitamin D3 in children and adults who have light skin. They advised that the diet should include 400–800 IU (10–20 mcg) per day from food fortified with vitamin D3 or supplements for populations at risk, such as those who spend little time outdoors, pregnant and lactating women, veiled women, those with dark skin, elderly, children, and infants.[399]

Vitamin D_3 creation within each person is complex beyond comprehension. This chapter has listed some of the many variables involved just in the amount of UVB radiation exposure for each person. Once the UVB rays enter the skin, the amount of vitamin D that is generated is then dependent on the amount of melanin in the skin, the amount of calcium and phosphorus in the body, the amount of cholesterol, a person's age and their own unique individual metabolism. To further complicate this already partial list of affecting variables, during the winter the amount that each person gradually converts from what they gained through the summer is also variable, with some people maintaining higher levels throughout the winter. This is why the studies, themselves, show disagreement as to what is the right amount of supplementation. Depending on where you live and how old you are, each person has to determine for themselves what is best for them in regards to sun exposure.

The best answer for each person is to test your vitamin D blood levels in late summer and late winter. These values will help you determine whether you are attaining a protective level in the summer, and how long it stays high enough to be protective for you through the winter. Based on these tests, you can decide if you need to supplement with vitamin D and if so, how much to take.

Most of the literature agrees that it is difficult to overdose with vitamin D supplementation. Studies suggest that taking between 1,000–5,000 IU (25–125 mcg) vitamin D_3 per day should be adequate without risking a toxic overload. This book provides a broad overview so that each individual can make the determination of what would be the right doses for them and their family. However, since the researchers themselves cannot agree on what is needed, each person needs to decide for themselves what plan of action to implement.

Chapter 17
Antioxidants – Mother Nature's Protective Sunscreens

In an article published in 2010, a researcher wrote: "The increasing incidence of skin cancer despite the use of externally applied sun protection strategies, alongside research showing that nutrients reduce photo-oxidative damage, suggest nutritional approaches could play a beneficial role in skin cancer prevention."[400]

Antioxidants: Prevent Skin Damage and Improve Skin Health

Antioxidants are components of the body's tumor protective cascade of compounds that prevent the changes that lead to cancer. Sunscreen manufacturers understanding that antioxidants reduce the number of ROS that form in the skin from their chemicals, as well as stabilize the sunscreen chemicals when they are exposed to sunlight, have been incorporating antioxidants into their formulas. The same antioxidant function sunscreen manufacturers are using in the formulas to reduce the ROS also applies to antioxidants that can be included in people's diets. Research has proven diets high in antioxidants provide the skin with natural protection from the sun's UV and IR radiation, as well as promote healthier skin. This is a natural way to protect the skin from sun damage. Most importantly, antioxidants are not foreign chemicals that can cause the harms identified in this book.

Researchers have determined that antioxidants are utilized very effectively by the body. In fact one research article described the process as: ". . . the skin possesses an elaborate antioxidant defense system to deal with UV-induced oxidative stress."[401]

Another wrote:

"A protection system has been developed by the human organism to combat the destructive action of free radicals. This protection system consists of antioxidant substances which form protection chains. Carotenoids, enzymes, and vitamins A, C, E, and D are the most important substances forming the aforementioned protective system in the human skin. The sum of the antioxidant substances in the body presents the antioxidant network."[402]

Antioxidants are the body's way of defending against the oxidative stress and potential DNA damage that can result in cancerous changes. Multiple studies show that a diet with high antioxidants combined with a low inflammatory affect, has been shown to reduce damaging effects from solar radiation. These antioxidants include not only vitamins C and E, and carotenoids, but also selenium, flavonoids, polyphenols, and plant oils.[403] The major radiation absorbing molecules in the skin (in addition to melanin) are amino acids and urocanic acids (metabolites of the amino acid histadine).[404] Antioxidants provide defense from UV radiation by protecting the skin in three ways.

1. Stopping the ROS from forming
2. Neutralizing ROS once they are formed
3. Reversing the damage that may be created in the skin

A one-year study on volunteers eating a diet rich in fruits and vegetables resulted in increased carotenoid levels in the skin. During the summer and fall months, an even greater increase was found in all volunteers. An additional important point demonstrated in this study was that even though the diet did not change, when there were stressors present in the volunteers lives, their carotenoid levels decreased. The stressors identified were fatigue, illness, smoking, and consumption of alcohol.[405]

In a 2006 study, researchers proved that diets with higher levels of antioxidants provide greater skin photoprotection, as well as improve skin health. The study involved two groups of women given cocoa powder with the antioxidant flavanol, in either high or low content. After 6 and 12 weeks of treatment, those in the high flavanol group showed significant photoprotection by demonstrating decreased skin reddening following UV radiation exposure. The antioxidant action of the flavanol also increased blood flow in all the skin layers, increased skin thickness, and skin hydration, while at the same time it resulted in a significant decrease of skin roughness and scaling.[406] These results show that antioxidants not only provide protection from the sun's rays, and therefore from photoaging, they reverse photoaging that may have taken place.

Antioxidants: Protect against IRA

Antioxidants are so protective against the IR spectrum of solar radiation that a 2011 study concluded:

"Nevertheless, at the present time, the best protection strategy against the destructive action of free radicals produced in human skin, subsequent to IR irradiation, is the high antioxidative network of the skin, which can be increased by means of antioxidant rich nutrition, for example, by fruit and vegetables, and topical application of cosmetic formulations containing a balanced mixture of antioxidants."

These researchers working with volunteers found that it takes between 1 to 2 days before the carotenoids return to the level that was in the skin prior to the IR radiation exposure, and the amount of time was dependent on the lifestyle of the volunteers. This led the researchers to recommend that it would be best to supplement with antioxidant fruits and vegetables prior to IR radiation exposure.[407]

Antioxidants: Protect the Total Body

High antioxidant intake is not only important for skin protection, free-radicals are thought to be responsible for the oxidative process and damage that result in age-related degeneration and disease. So, the added benefit is that they are not only very helpful for sun protection, by protecting from oxidation damage in all the systems of the body, they also reduce the progression of disease, and aging as well. Antioxidants can help reduce oxidative damage in the heart, liver, and testicles, where they protect sperm and ultimately fertility.[408] Antioxidants provide such health benefits by reducing ROS throughout the body it behooves everyone to reduce the stressors in their lives that decrease antioxidant levels, as fewer antioxidants result in decreasing the body's ability to withstand the damage that ROS can create.[409]

Antioxidants that Are Proven to Provide Sunscreen Protection

There are many classes of antioxidants. This chapter cannot list them all, but highlights those that have been studied in relation to protection from UV radiation. Listed below are some of the main groups of antioxidants that have been investigated.

Anthocyanins
Beta-carotene
Carotenoids
Flavonoids
Polyphenols
Stilbenes
Tocopherols
Tocotrienols

Antioxidant Oxygen Radical Absorbance Capacity (ORAC)

Due to antioxidants many benefits throughout the body, the U.S. Department of Agriculture has developed a system that measures foods and supplements according to their effectiveness to neutralize free radicals. Termed the Oxygen Radical Absorbance Capacity (ORAC), they have assigned a value that reflects their antioxidant capacity: the greater the antioxidant activity the food or supplement supplies, the higher the assigned ORAC value. Throughout the remainder of this book, the ORAC values that have been measured will be next to the foods and supplements (e.g., rosemary, dried 165,000) that are discussed. The ORAC values are based on a volume of 3 1/2 oz. (100 g) and the foods will be listed in most cases in descending order of activity. As of the beginning of 2011, not all foods have been tested, so some foods will have no value next to them. The Website address for an updated list can be found in Appendix A.[410]

Antioxidants Work Together in Synergistic Harmony

There are antioxidants that are stable by themselves, such as vitamin C, vitamin E, and carnosic acid (from rosemary), which all exhibit a protective role from the oxidative stress of UV radiation.

Some antioxidants need other vitamins for stability. These include the carotenoids, like lycopene and beta-carotene, which need the protection of the antioxidant vitamin E in order for them to function as antioxidants. Vitamin E does this by increasing the stability and cellular uptake of lycopene.[411]

Vitamin E, Vitamin C, CoQ10, and Carotenoids

Vitamin E, vitamin C, and carotenoids function as antioxidants by reacting with ROS free radicals. Vitamin C acts in the watery portion of body fluids, and vitamin E and carotenoids, beta-carotene, lycopene, and oxycarotenoids (e.g., zeaxanthin and lutein), act in the fatty portion of the cellular compartments. Vitamin E consists of a collection of tocopherols that provide the majority of antioxidant protection against free radicals in biological membranes, reducing DNA damage and cancerous changes. Vitamin C and CoQ10 support the antioxidant activity of vitamin E by regenerating it back to its antioxidant form when the body has utilized it to neutralize free radicals.[412]

Direct Acting Antioxidants

Antioxidants can work directly to neutralize ROS so they can be harmlessly removed from the body. Direct antioxidants include lycopene, lutein, beta-carotene, and quercetin, which are found in fruits and vegetables.[413]

Indirect Acting Antioxidants

Glucosinolates

There are nutrients that act indirectly to activate the body's own antioxidant and detoxification systems. Glucosinolates belong to the group of indirect antioxidants. They are part of a cascade of antioxidant activity that repeatedly recycles throughout the body to provide continuous protection for 3 to 4 days after eating glucosinolate containing foods.

The enzyme pathways the liver uses to cleanse toxins from the body are assisted by glucosinolates. The foods containing the highest level of the glucosinolates are broccoli sprouts, cauliflower sprouts, and less high are alfalfa sprouts. The sprouts have the highest concentration because glucosinolates are what the plant itself uses to protect its young growth.[413]

Found in:
Broccoli sprouts – highest
Cauliflower sprouts – highest
Alfalfa sprouts
Cruciferous vegetables
Broccoli
Cauliflower
Bok choy
Brussels sprouts
Cabbage
Kale

Polyphenols

Polyphenols are the most abundant antioxidants in our diets, and several thousand have been identified. Listed among their many varied functions is their ability to act as protective agents against UV light.[414] Foods with polyphenols are easy to recognize as they are the antioxidants that give fruits and vegetables their bright colored reds, yellows, and purples. Of the polyphenols, the flavonoids are the most abundant in our diets. Polyphenols are generally higher in fruits than in vegetables, however, their diverse structures as well as lack of standardized testing methods make their content in foods difficult to estimate. Tests on laboratory animals show that the polyphenols absorb all the UVB radiation along with part of the UVA, as well as UVC radiation. By protecting from the adverse affects UV wavelengths can create, polyphenols reduce oxidative stress, inflammation, and DNA damage, which results in the reduction of the risk of skin cancers. The polyphenols in green tea are readily absorbed and studies show they rapidly remove or repair damage done to DNA by UVB radiation. The conclusion from the research is routine consumption or topical application of polyphenols can provide efficient protection from UV radiation.[415] For those who would like a detailed breakdown of the various categories of polyphenols and the foods that contain them, they are listed in Appendix A.

Specific Antioxidants

The rest of this chapter lists the many antioxidants that provide sun protection and the foods that have them in high concentrations.

Organic Foods

In reducing the possibility of estrogenic disruption from sunscreens, it is also important not to ingest pesticides as they also have estrogenic properties and can cause hormone disruption.[416] So, when adding or increasing these foods in your diet, do include organic as much as possible.

Aloe vera

Scientists have confirmed that aloe vera contains antioxidants, along with many other nutrients. Aloe vera is also recorded as being used by the Egyptians to protect their skin from the sun, even Cleopatra is said to have used it on her skin.[417]

Found in:
Many lotions are available that contain aloe vera.
Plants can be grown to harvest the leaves, which can be cut open so the gel from inside the leaf can be placed directly on the skin as well as the hair.

Amino acid: histadine

Histadine provides UV protection.   In addition to melanin, histadine is a major absorber of UV radiation in the skin. It not only protects in the skin, it also is involved in tissue repair.

Found in:
Protein foods
Meat
Poultry
Fish
Dairy

Grains
  Wheat
  Rice
  Rye

Amino acid: L-ergothioneine
  L-ergothioneine is an integral part of the antioxidative defense system of the skin that not only prevents oxidative damage but also may facilitate DNA repair in cells that have been exposed to UV radiation.[418] It is an amino acid with great antioxidant capacity that is manufactured by fungi. Mushrooms contain 40 times more than other foods.

Found in:[419]
Mushrooms
  Shiitake, dried   800   ORAC value
  Maitake   700
  Oyster   700
  King Oyster
Others
  Wheat germ
  Chicken livers

Anthocyanins
  Anthocyanins protect against solar radiation and are in many foods. Cosmetic manufacturers adding anthocyanin extracts from the purple sweet potato to cosmetic cream found they absorb 46% of the UV radiation, more of the UVB compared with UVA.[420]

Found in:
Red and blue colored fruit and vegetables
  Red grapes – highest   1,800   ORAC value
  Eggplant – highest   900
  Elderberries   14,700

Blueberries, raw wild	10,000
Plums	8,000
Raspberries, raw	5,100
Pomegranates	4,500
Red cabbage, raw	2,500
Chocolate, Tea, Coffee	
Baking chocolate, unsweetened	50,000
Cocoa (mixed powder)	485
Green tea	1,300
Black tea	1,100
White tea	300
Coffee	

Coffee lovers will appreciate the outcome of studies that show caffeine prevents UV cell damage (even in the corneal layer of the eye).[421]   Coffee and tea provide 85–100% UV protection, while cocoa provides 50% UV protection. However, studies have varying results, with some finding caffeine "alone" provided no protection, while others found it does offer protection in the form of caffeine sodium benzoate, rather than as just caffeine. Based on these studies, it appears that extracting the caffeine for use by itself does not provide the protection researchers identify when utilizing the whole tea, coffee, or cocoa liquid.[422] As with everything, it is balance, as too much caffeine can led to cell death.

Astaxanthin

Astaxanthin, a carotenoide, demonstrates that it provides 500 times stronger antioxidant protection than vitamin E, and is 10 times stronger than vitamin A (betacarotene). In relation to the effects of sunlight exposure, it increases immune system function, and reduces the inflammation that leads to sunburn. For those who have stayed out in the sun too long, astaxanthin can reduce the pain and swelling associated with sunburn.[423]

Found in:[424]
Red colored fish and shellfish
   Crab
   Crawfish
   Crustaceans
   Krill
   Lobster
   Rainbow trout
   Salmon
   Shrimp
Red and orange colored vegetables
   Red peppers   800   ORAC value
   Carrots   700
Microalgae
Yeast

It is available as a supplement.

Carnosine

Carnosine is a naturally occurring amino acid (a combination of alanine and histadine) that decreases as people age. Found in the muscles, brain and nervous system, carnosine protects and stabilizes cell membranes. Carnosine and homocarnosine have antioxidant effects that protect DNA from damage. A 2010 study identified that carnosine, and compounds related to it, may be protective when there are pathological conditions that create DNA damage that can lead to the degenerative changes seen in neurodegenerative disorders.[425] As a result, carnosine has been studied in Alzheimer's patients where it has been shown to decrease and reverse cell damage.[426] It is also found to be helpful with cataracts, and Parkinson's disease.[427]

Found in:
Protein-rich foods
  Beef
  Poultry
  Pork
  Milk
  Eggs
  Cheese

It is available as a supplement.

Vegetarians and the elderly need to make sure their diet includes an ample supply of proteins. If their diet does not, carnosine should be taken as a supplement to protect cells from oxidation damage.[428]

Carnosic acid
    Carnosic acid (a polyphenol) acts as an antioxidant. It also helps increase the production of glutathione, which is an important antioxidant used throughout the body (see glutathione below for details).[429]

Found in:

Rosemary, dried	165,000 ORAC value
Sage, ground	120,000
Sage, fresh	32,000

Ferulic acid
    Ferulic acid is a natural component of plant cell walls. It is currently being studied for UV protection of the skin, prevention of cancer in many organs, as a cholesterol and lipid balancer protecting the heart, as well as protection of the brain in preventing Alzheimer's disease. Body-builders also use it to repair muscles. It already is being incorporated, along with other antioxidants, into lotions formulated as sunscreens.[430]

Found in:[431]
Brown rice – greatest source
Whole wheat
Oats

Artichokes	9,400	ORAC value
Peanuts, raw	3,200	
Apples	2,500	
Oranges	2,000	
Pineapples	600	
Coffee		

It is available as a supplement.

Ferulic acid is part of the gamma oryzanol plant complex discussed below.

Gamma oryzanol

Derived from rice bran oil, gamma oryzanol is a mixture of plant chemicals that have antioxidant function. This is what was in the plants that Egyptians used for their sun protection 1,000s of years ago. Today's chemists have proven that it does protect against oxidation in the skin. This antioxidant activity was confirmed in a study published in the *Journal of Agriculture and Food Chemistry* in 2011. They looked at the antioxidant and free radical scavenging activity of pigmented rice bran and determined gamma oryzanol was the major antioxidant. The rice bran also contained anthocyanins, alpha-tocopherol (vitamin E), and phenolic acids. They further concluded that by adding 5% black rice bran to wheat flour when making bread, the supplemented bread had a marked increase in the free radical scavenging and antioxidant activity when compared to wheat bread without the added rice bran.[432] In addition, it also has the added benefit of reducing cholesterol and lipids in the blood.[433]

Found in:[434]

Rice bran   24,300   ORAC value
Grains – especially high in wheat bran
Some fruits and vegetables

It is available as a supplement.

Glutathione

Glutathione is one of the body's most important antioxidants that helps protect against free radical damage in the skin, as well as in the brain. Since glutathione cannot be taken orally, as it is destroyed by the stomach, the body needs to manufacture it from the amino acids: glycine; cysteine; and glutamate. However, selenium, sulfur, and vitamin D are also necessary parts and must be available for the process to take place. This is another benefit of making sure you have enough vitamin D from either sun exposure or from taking it as a supplement. Glutathione is also too large to enter the cell, so the cells themselves need to assemble glutathione within each cell. To make adequate amounts, diets have to include all the components the cells require to make their own glutathione.

Based on its antioxidant capabilities, researchers are looking at glutathione in relation to Alzheimer's disease and its ability to reduce oxidative stress. Oxidative stress has been identified as a key factor involved in Alzheimer's disease, as free radical oxidative damage has been found to be extensive in the brains of Alzheimer's patients.[435] Studies are demonstrating glutathione helps reduce the oxidative stress that appears to play a role in the development and progression of the Alzheimer's disease.[436]

Found in:

Strawberries	4,300	ORAC value
Asparagus	2,150	
Peach	1,900	
Grapefruit	1,600	
Spinach	1,600	
Potatoes	1,600	
Squash Zucchini	400	
Cantaloupe	300	
Watermelon	100	

Foods that increase glutathione levels and activity:

Rosemary, dried	165,000
Spinach	1,500
Avocado	1,370
Broccoli	1,350

Dairy – cheese (cottage and ricotta),
    eggs, yogurt, milk
Grains – oats, wheat germ, granola

Nutrients that increase glutathione levels and activity:[437]
    Fish oil
    Alpha lipoic acid
    SAMe
    Selenium (Brazil nuts, meats, sea foods).
    Vitamin E
    Vitamin C
    Vitamin Bs – B12, B6, B2 (riboflavin), and folate
        (sunflower seeds, green leafy vegetables, avocados)
    Milk thistle

Sulfur in adequate concentration is necessary for glutathione functioning.

Sulfur rich foods:

Garlic	5,500 ORAC value
Broccoli	2,800
Cabbage red	2,400
Asparagus	2,100
Onions	2,000
Cabbage green	500
Watercress	
Kale	
Brussels sprouts	
Turnips	

Amino acids are necessary for glutathione functioning.
Whey protein contains amino acids [undenatured has highest source of cysteine].

Quercetin

A flavonoid polyphenol, studies have shown that quercetin protects against UVB radiation in mice.[438]

Found in:[439]
Bright colored fruits and vegetables
Green leafy vegetables
Capers
Onions
Garlic
Cocoa

It is available as a supplement.

Resveratrol

Since resveratrol demonstrates antioxidant activity, researchers exposed epidermal skin cells to UVA wavelengths and found that resveratrol protects from ROS generation, increases cell viability, and increases the activity of antioxidant enzymes. These results show that resveratrol provides natural protection of skin cells from UVA induced radiation damage.[440]

Found in:[441]

Blueberries, wild raw	10,000	ORAC value
Blackberries	4,000	
Peanuts raw	3,200	
Red grapes	1,800	

It is available as a supplement in a concentrated form.

Foods with Proven High Antioxidant Action

Avocados

After identifying many antioxidants and compounds in avocados, researchers incubated human cells with avocado extracts. Even at very low concentrations, the human cells showed antioxidant protection with reduced signs of oxidative stress, along with less DNA and cellular damage — a protective effect that lasted over 12 hours.[442]

Avocados	1,900	ORAC value

Broccoli sprouts

Broccoli sprouts are high in several beneficial antioxidants. They are not only high in glucosinolates; they are also rich in glucoraphanin, which transforms into the isothiocyanate, sulforaphane. Sulforaphane activates an enzyme that protects the cells from cancerous changes. Researchers have found whether glucoraphanin is applied topically or given orally, the incidence of tumors in mice after UV radiation exposure is reduced by 25%, the number of tumors reduced by 47%, along with a 70% reduction in their size.[443]

Cantaloupe extract: superoxide dismutase (SOD)

Cantaloupe extract contains superoxide dismutase (SOD), which is an antioxidant that protects against UV radiation damage. Due to this action, SOD has been incorporated into hair and skin products as protection against UV radiation damage.[444]

Goji berry juice

The goji berry, *Lycium barbarum*, has antioxidant effects. Mice, given 5% goji berry juice showed significantly reduced inflammatory sunburn reaction. The researchers concluded their results suggest that consumption of this juice could provide additional photoprotection, as various dilutions of goji berry juice showed dose-dependent protection against the immunosuppression that solar radiation can create.[445]

Goji berry juice, raw   3,300   ORAC value

Tea: drinking or skin application

The best support you can provide your skin to protect it from solar radiation of any wavelength is to supply the body with the antioxidative elements it uses in its natural protection processes. This applies to both taking the antioxidants in through the diet, as well as applying them directly to the skin.

Studies confirm that green tea, whether taken internally as a drink, or applied to the skin, is very protective and prevents tumor growth in mice. It was found to decrease the changes that result in melanoma, as well as the basal and squamous cell carcinomas.[446] Another study on rat cells showed it protects against ROS and cell death.[447]

Teas:

Green tea	1,300 ORAC value
Black tea	1,100
White tea	300

Spices

Their high ORAC values show spices have far greater antioxidant capacity than other foods.[448] The problem, however, is that they are usually used in very small quantities. If you have not used spices liberally in the past, now may be the time to start adding them to most of the dishes you eat.

Cloves, ground	290,000 ORAC value
Oregano, dried	175,000
Rosemary, dried	165,000
Thyme, dried	157,000
Cinnamon, ground	130,000
Turmeric, ground	127,000
Vanilla beans	122,000
Sage, ground	120,000
Szechwan pepper, dried	118,000
Parsley, dried	74,000
Nutmeg, ground	70,000
Basil, dried	61,000
Cumin seed	50,000
Curry powder	49,000
Ginger, ground	39,000
Pepper, black	34,000
Mustard seeds	29,000
Marjoram, fresh	27,000
Thyme, fresh	27,000
Chili powder	24,000

Tarragon, fresh	16,000
Oregano, fresh	14,000
Basil, fresh	4,800

Antioxidants with Proven IR Protection

Research has proven there are chemicals that protect against IR radiation. These include:[449]

Genistein (soybeans)
Vitamin C
Flavonoids
N-acetylcysteine

Antioxidant UV Protection Diet
Strengthens the Immune System and Protects from Cancer

A fully balanced antioxidant diet will lead to a strong immune system. It is clear that when the immune system is strong, the body's antioxidants will hunt out and eliminate cells that have been damaged. Creating a healthy immune system will not only provide protection from skin cancers, but may also protect from cancers throughout the body.

Antioxidants are the components the body uses for its own DNA repair systems. Having a healthy repair system is critical, as it has been identified that 50% of basal cell carcinomas are not created by UV radiation. This was determined because the basal cells did not have the UV signature they would have if the cancer was caused by solar radiation.[450]

Is Anti-inflammatory

An anti-inflammation diet needs to include sources that are rich in omega-3 fatty acids, which a study in mice showed they reduce UV radiation immune suppression and cancer. The study identified that it is the eicosapentaenoic acid (EPA) in the omega-3 rather than the docosahexaenoic acid (DHA) that resulted in the protection.[451] This is in contrast to the omega-6 fatty acids that do not demonstrate this protection and may even increase the changes that can result in increased risk of melanomas and skin cancers.[452] These results are confirmed in a study where a high ratio of omega-3 compared to omega-6 showed a lower risk of both melanoma and squamous cell carcinoma.[453]

Reverses Photoaging
    Incorporating a high antioxidant and anti-inflammatory diet has another advantage as studies are proving they reverse and repair damage that may have been caused by staying out in the sun too long.[454] Just as with the experiments that showed the whole coffee or tea provided more protection than the extracted caffeine, so eating the whole plant containing the antioxidants will provide far better protection than just taking the selected extracts, such as those found in supplements. A diet full of antioxidant rich foods will not only provide UV protection, it will also benefit every organ system in the body, providing the best health and least deterioration as we grow older. For the complete list of antioxidants identified in this chapter, see Appendix A.

After Sun Protection
Olive Oil Provides Healing Antioxidant Activity in Skin after Sun Exposure
    Olive oil and olives contain several antioxidants that are shown to reduce the effects of oxidative stress and readily cross cell membranes, providing cellular protection. This aspect of cell protection is one reason it is theorized to provide the helpful benefits for the cardiovascular system that is seen in the Mediterranean diet.[455]
    In fact, olive oil has many beneficial qualities. A study published in 2010 describes that in addition to being an antioxidant, its many actions include being anti-inflammatory, antiatherogenic (reduces plaque in arteries), anti-cancer, antibacterial, antiviral, as well as reduces blood lipids (HDL, LDL, cholesterol) and sugar.[456] When

olive oil is applied to the skin after sun exposure, it provides the same protection for the oxidative damage caused by the sun. Researchers conclude their results suggest that daily topical use of super virgin olive oil after sun bathing may delay and reduce UV-induced skin cancer development in human skin.[457]

Tea: Topical Application

Applying tea after sun exposure provides protection in several ways. Investigators applying either white or green tea found that it protects the skin from UV created immunosuppression.[458]   Several studies have also demonstrated that the polyphenols found in green tea are beneficial in several ways in protecting the skin from cancers. In addition to reducing the ROS and DNA damage, they reverse the inflammatory response, and repair damage that may have occurred due to the exposure.[459]   Indeed, topical application to the skin is confirmed in a study published in 2008 where researchers identified the damaging effects that can result from IR radiation in human skin are inhibited by the topical application of antioxidants.[460]

Making a heavily brewed cup of black tea using several tea bags, cooling it with ice, and applying it with a cloth or paper towel to the skin is not only healing, it is also very soothing after sun exposure. Applying it reduces the reddening and pain of sunburn and helps promote tanning of the skin.

Antioxidant Diet Provides Protective New Lifestyle

After ingestion, antioxidants are distributed to the tissues exposed to light — the skin and eyes — where they provide protection for the cells. Some research is demonstrating that protection can occur within 2 to 3 days on increasing antioxidants in the diet.[461]   Other researchers demonstrated a 50% reduction in skin reddening reaction after 6 weeks and a 70% reduction after 12 weeks of high-flavanol cocoa.[462]

Chapter 18
Sun Protective Clothing

Our ancestors may have been smarter than we are, because historically, styles of clothing through the centuries have covered the majority of the body. At the turn of the 20th century, the Victorian Era of clothing had bathing suits that covered the body down to the elbows and knees, and often completely covering the legs. Even men's swim suits included tops that covered their chest, stomach, and back. Women's clothing covered them to their wrists and to their ankles, and they routinely wore hats and gloves. So it has only been since the 1920s that their has been less and less covering of the body with swim suits and clothes, creating the need to be concerned about the excess exposure to the sun's rays on the skin.[463]

Cloth itself naturally blocks many, if not most, of the sun's radiation. There are several general guidelines that can be used in the selection of clothing for protection during excess exposure. The tighter the cloth's weave, the more it shields the sun's rays. Also, synthetic fabrics have a greater blocking affect than natural fabrics, such as cotton. Additionally, the darker the color, the more protection it provides.

Fabric can be submitted to laboratories that test for the amount of UV radiation that it allows through. There are several scales that are utilized to determine the amount of UV radiation allowed through the material being tested. One is called Biological Dosimetry (BD), where they perform two types of measurements: one stationary BD in the laboratory; and the other they call real life testing or mobile subject BD testing.

The other rating scale that has been developed to classify a fabric's level of protection is similar to SPF for sunscreen lotions. Called the

Ultraviolet Protection Factor (UPF), it specifies the amount of time the clothing can protect from solar radiation, with a UPF value of 1 equal to protection from approximately 10 minutes of sunlight. The rating ranks the fabric on a scale from 15 to 50, with 50 providing the ultimate amount of UV protection as shown in Table 11.[464]

Table 11.   **UPF Rating System**

Rating	UV Rays Blocked	Protection Level
15+	93.3-95.8%	Good
25+	95.9-97.4%	Very good
40+	more than 97.5%	Excellent
50+	Considered the ultimate UV sun protection.	

These different methods of testing each provide significantly different results as to how much of the UV radiation is blocked.[465] As sunlight is diffuse and more scattered and absorbed by the fabric compared to artificial radiation, UPF values obtained by measurements in real exposure situations are usually higher than those obtained with artificial radiation, and could account for the discrepancy between laboratory testing and field measurements.[466] Even though there are discrepancies over how much UV is blocked whether one method of testing is performed versus another, it appears that the UPF rating is becoming the dominant labeling preference.

Manufacturers are creating fabrics utilizing a tighter weave knit to deliberately block out the UV radiation for prevention of skin cancer formation, light sensitivity disorders, and premature skin aging. One called UV-Cut fabric has been created to provide a longer period of protection and is rated according to the first 3 levels of the UPF system that is listed above to indicate the extent of UV protection. In addition to blocking UV, it also importantly reduces thermal transmission (keeps the heat out).

More recently, one manufacturer of UV protective clothing has utilized fluorescent particles to reduce UV rays, while amplifying the yellow light rays, and allowing infrared rays (IR) through.[467] Since as shown in Chapter 15, IR can lead to the same type of damage as UV, this does not appear to be an answer that would protect from the cell damage and photoaging that IR radiation can cause.

TiO_2 and ZnO Nanoparticle Cloth

Some manufactures today are creating UV-protective clothing by incorporating titanium and zinc oxides into the materials they are developing. The average size of the ZnO nanoparticles they are using is estimated to be 38 nm.[468] Research shows that ZnO nanoparticles are more abrasive than the larger bulk ZnO. This results in their being more antimicrobial due to the mechanical damage they inflict on the cell membrane. Due to the antibacterial nature of TiO_2 nanoparticles, polyester with TiO_2 nanoparticles is being promoted for incorporation not only into clothing to be worn in the sun, but also into underwear, socks, and carpets. Furthermore, manufacturers are saying TiO_2 nanoparticle cotton can be utilized in medicine as bed sheets, surgical clothes, doctors' uniforms, or patient clothing, and for general use as clothes in the food industry, bedding, and furniture fabrics.[469]

TiO_2 nanoparticles are also being incorporated into fabrics due to their ability to eliminate stains when the fabric is exposed to sunlight. The sizes that are being utilized for this are nanoparticles that are only 4–5 nm, or 0.004–0.005 microns, far, far smaller than the human sweat pore size of 15–80 microns.[470] This means they are very capable of gaining entrance through the skin from contact with cloth that is impregnated with them. The sun works very well, by itself, at removing stains in fabric that has not been impregnated with TiO_2 nanoparticles, making this increased risk unnecessary.

The ZnO nanoparticles that are impregnated into cloth do wash out into our wastewater systems during the laundering process, as their antimicrobial affect is lost after 20 washes.[471] This means that ZnO nanoparticles must be washed away in the water that will eventually be released back into the rivers and waterways, and ultimately into the oceans where they have been proven to kill plankton. Also, hospitals would have to purchase bedding and uniforms on a continual basis if they were bought with the idea that they were antimicrobial, as they would no longer possess that quality after 20 washes.

Nanoparticles: Hazard to Humans and Ecosystem

With all of these new ways of introducing nanoparticles into our environment, it is important to keep in mind that all of the possibilities of harm these tiny particles can inflict would apply to cloth that is impregnated with them. Due to their abrasive nature, TiO_2 nanoparticle skin exposure can lead to irritation. Also, researchers have found that chronic exposure to nanoparticles can lead to deterioration of pulmonary lung function. Some workers in TiO_2 nanoparticle manufacturing plants show signs of lung fibrosis from breathing in the nanoparticles. The recommended safety guidelines for those who work with titanium dioxide nanoparticles are listed below.

"PERSONAL HYGIENE PROCEDURES

If titanium dioxide collects on the skin, workers should wash the affected areas with soap and water.

Clothing contaminated with titanium dioxide should be removed, and provisions should be made for the safe removal of the chemical from the clothing.

A worker who handles titanium dioxide should thoroughly wash hands, forearms, and face with soap and water before eating, using tobacco products, using toilet facilities, or applying cosmetics.

Workers should not eat, drink, use tobacco products, or apply cosmetics in areas where titanium dioxide is handled, processed, or stored."[472]

Why would it be safe to incorporate TiO_2 nanoparticles into the sunscreens, cosmetics, clothing, and medical bedding and uniforms when these types of precautions are recommended for the workers where the nanoparticles are being manufactured?

Flame Retardant Polybrominated Diphenyl Ether Regulations

Can we also learn from the government mandated use of the flame retardant Polybrominated Diphenyl Ether (PDBE)? It certainly falls into another "law of unintended consequences." Even though concern over the health safety and the possibility that the PDBEs may be linked to sudden infant death syndrome (SIDS), researchers in 1995 stated their evidence did not support the causal relationship and that the benefit of fire safety outweighed the potential for any risk.[473]

However, 15 years later there has finally been enough accumulated evidence that the flame retardants do pose a health hazard, resulting in 15 more years of exposing our infants and children to these chemicals, and releasing them to the entire ecosystem. One study concluded with the words:

"As a consequence of substantial, long-term usage, polybrominated diphenyl ethers (PBDEs) have contaminated humans, wildlife, and abiotic (environmental) matrices around the world."[474]

There is now concern over the amount of the flame retardant chemical, polybrominated diphenyl ether (PBDE), found in children's blood in the United States. As a result of the drive to protect children from the potential hazard of fire, flame retardants have been incorporated into many items that surround our children, including the mattresses they sleep on for a good portion of every 24 hours, during their most crucial periods of early development. Studies are showing that the amount found in their blood parallels the amount found in the dust of their homes, so they are now breathing them in on a continuous basis, and are particularly high in California residents due to their strict flammability laws.[475]   This is alarming as studies are also revealing that flame retardant causes neurodevelopmental impairments and lowered IQs.[476]

On April 12, 2010 the concern over the harm to our children prompted two members of the U.S. House of Representatives to open an inquiry regarding the health and environmental impact of the flame retardants.[477]   In a 2010 article published in *Reviews on Environmental Health*, researchers summed up the far reaching effects of flame retardant use.

"Since the 1970s, an increasing number of regulations have expanded the use of brominated and chlorinated flame retardants. Many of these chemicals are now recognized as global contaminants and are associated with adverse health effects in animals and humans, including endocrine and thyroid disruption, immunotoxicity, reproductive toxicity, cancer, and adverse effects on fetal and child development and neurologic function. Some flame retardants such as polybrominated diphenyl ethers (PBDEs) have been banned or voluntarily phased out by manufacturers because of their environmental persistence and toxicity, only to be replaced by other organohalogens of unknown toxicity."[478]

Everything we use eventually finds its way back to our environment and impacts the earth's entire ecosystem. This is clearly shown by the fact that birds throughout America and Europe are now found to have the flame retardant chemicals in their bodies.

Flame Retardants and Sunscreens Now Ubiquitous

The drive to protect children from fire has resulted in the unintended consequences of hurting them. Let us not allow this to be the result of the continued use of the UV sunscreens and UV protective cloth and clothing, which will impact millions more children than have already been impacted if we do not remove them from the market.

Looking at the biochemistry of nanoparticles and that they are capable of entering inside the cell nucleus causing disrupted cell division, we can protect our children now by not using nanoparticle sunscreens, nor purchasing clothing that has been impregnated with nanoparticles. Since it is shown the nanoparticles come off with water in the laundry, it makes sense they would come off onto the skin as a result of sweating or swimming. Avoid materials coated with these metals, as tightly woven cloth, by itself, can provide excellent protection without exposing all life on the planet to the harm the increased use of TiO_2 and ZnO nanoparticles can cause.

Chapter 19
Cosmetics and Body Lotions

As of the date of this writing, this chapter is necessarily extremely short. It is very difficult today to find make-up and any type of product to be used on the body that does not contain a sunscreen chemical or nanoparticle of some type. Many make-up foundations and lipsticks contain TiO_2 nanoparticles. However, this leads consumers to a false sense of protection as TiO_2 nanoparticles do not cover as much of the spectrum of the sun's rays compared to ZnO. In fact a study published in 2010 in the *American Journal of Clinical Dermatology* concluded: "Hence, TiO_2 cannot be considered a substitute for avobenzone or ZnO in providing high levels of UVA protection to human skin."[479] Yet, many make up and lipstick formulations contain only TiO_2 nanoparticles and are promoted and marketed that they provide protection from the sun.

Even though avobenzone has not been shown to be as great an endocrine disrupting chemical (EDC), it is not an answer either. Since it is not stable in sunlight, in order for it to act as a UV filter for any length of time other chemicals must be included in the formulations.[480] This not only results in greater possibility of skin penetration, but also of harmful combinations as many of the other chemicals it is being mixed with show they are EDCs or are nanoparticles.

To date, we have not identified a manufacturer of a line of body products that does not contain chemical or nanoparticle sunscreen ingredients. We will keep working on identifying these and will make the information available in our continually on-going newsletter. Information on obtaining this valuable resource guide is provided at the end of the book.

Chapter 20
The Sunscreen Market

The evidence of increasing skin cancer and melanoma is very clear now, and reveals that the partial protection that sunscreens have provided has caused more harm than not using sunscreen at all and staying in the sun less. As sunscreen manufacturers have realized that sunscreens are not protecting the skin in the ways that they have been promoted to do, newer sunscreen chemicals are now rapidly being incorporated into sunscreen formulations to provide the broad spectrum of filtering out both UVB and UVA rays, which they now know should have always been incorporated into every sunscreen from the beginning.[481]

At the time of this publication, safety reviews of new products primarily only include contact sensitivity data (i.e., whether they create an allergic reaction). Unfortunately, when they make it past this hurdle, they are concluded to be safe. These new chemicals, however, are where the older ones were when they were made into sunscreen formulas before all the safety testing was completed on them. Benzophenone has been used since the 1980s, yet the majority of the studies identifying that it is an endocrine disrupting EDC did not get published until after 2000, and the studies proving disruption to thyroid hormones were not published until 2009. It is clear that it takes 20 to 30 years of studying each new chemical before all potential impacts can be analyzed and clarified. Therefore, these new products should be kept off the market until generational studies on mice or rats, as well as their impact on fish, coral, and plankton, have been fully evaluated and results from these studies are incorporated into the final assessment of whether the new chemicals are truly safe or not.

This chapter lists some of the newest chemicals and ideas for protecting the skin, along with the reasons why they should not be adopted until more is known about the impact their long-term use will have on humans and the environment.

New Untested Frontiers in Sunscreen Technology
Chemicals
Ecamsule

Manufacturers have been incorporating this relatively newer chemical, ecamsule, into what they are terming broad spectrum protection. There have not been enough studies to clarify whether this new chemical will cause the same hormonal disruption as found in the sunscreen chemicals that have been utilized to date.

Osmolytes

Osmolytes are utilized by cells to control cell volumes, and are part of what the cell utilizes in its defense against environmental stressors. Due to their demonstrating protection against detrimental UV effects, the osmolytes taurine13 and ectoine14 are already included in several commercially available sunscreens.[482]

Physical Encapsulation

Sunscreen manufacturers are working on encapsulating sunscreen ingredients inside liposome or silica shells. They theorize that this would reduce the possibility of skin irritation or allergic reactions as the chemicals would not come in direct contact with the skin. Another advantage they believe would be that the encapsulated material would scatter more UV rays, so less of the chemical would be necessary to achieve the same amount of protection. Unfortunately, this is still utilizing the same chemical sunscreens that have been shown to produce harm.[483] Also, encapsulating within silica shells has shown to produce more toxicity. See Chapter 13 for more detail regarding this technology.

This encapsulation technology is being investigated for the sunscreen chemical avobenzone combined with the cinnamate EHMC, which researchers state would limit the potential toxicological risks involved with exposing the body to the chemicals.[484] This makes no sense, if a chemical is a potential toxin, it should not be used at all. If they are concerned about limiting toxic risk, how can they measure the degree to which this technology would limit the risk?

Artificial Hormone Induction

Researchers are investigating the use of melanocyte stimulating hormone (MSH) to induce the melanocytes that are in the epidermal layer of the skin to increase the amount of melanin.[485] Since melanin absorbs UV radiation, it is the body's way of providing natural built-in protection from solar radiation. However, a melanocyte stimulating hormone would not be an innocent bystander, because this hormone influences many areas of the body in addition to the skin. Melanin involves other hormones as it is stimulated by the hormones adrenocorticotropic hormone (ACTH), estrogens, and progesterone.[486] Melanin also impacts mucus membranes in the nose and lungs, and is involved with the hypothalamus in creating melanin and endorphins. It would be very difficult to determine what far reaching effects could occur from artificially raising MSH levels in the body.[487]

Bacteria Products & DNA Technology

Bacteria Enzyme Delivered Intercellularly

A DNA repair enzyme that is found in bacteria is being investigated. When delivered intracellularly, it speeds up the repair of DNA in human cells and has been found to be protective against basal cell carcinoma and actinic keratosis (rough, scaly patch of skin).[488]

Bacterial Mycosporines and Mycosporine-like Amino Acids

Researchers have found that cyanobacteria (blue-green algae) make small-molecule sunscreens called mycosporines and mycosporine-like amino acids (MAAs) that combat UV exposure by absorbing the harmful rays. They have been able to identify the genes and enzymes involved in the biosynthesis of these sunscreening molecules.[489]   It could be that these may one day be a safe answer to protecting our skin without harming ourselves or the environment.

DNA Repair Enzymes and Reversing Skin Aging

Enzymes that the body uses to repair DNA damage are being studied to see if this type of technique could provide therapeutic interventions for aging skin in the future.[490]   Experimenting with encapsulating them and applying them directly to the skin is demonstrating that they can repair DNA that has been damaged by UVB radiation.[491]   However, they are not proving to be beneficial in preventing melanoma.[492] Since they are enzymes, they would not stay in their active form without encapsulating them. Again, please see the previous section on encapsulation presented in this chapter.

Antioxidants

One antioxidant that has been adopted by sunscreen manufacturers is *Cassia alata* leaf extract. Over the years, this has been used as an anti-fungal agent, and has been verified that it is also anti-bacterial, as well as has laxative properties.[493]

It is an excellent antioxidant for protection of the skin, so it is being incorporated into some of the sunscreen formulations that are available today. However, it is being included in products that contain many of the chemicals that are harmful, so these products should still be avoided.

IR Protection

IR protecting formulations present a whole new field of investigations, as IR is only beginning to be addressed in sunscreens. It is very difficult to design a chemical that would block IR, so researchers are having to turn to what they call secondary photoprotection, which utilizes "active" agents that will interfere with or counteract the changes that IR radiation induces and leads to DNA damage in skin cells.

Alphabet Soup

Needing to stop IR radiation at the cellular level means that scientists are researching new levels of biochemicals functioning at the level of the cell. The compounds they are looking at have so many letters, reading the research regarding them is like looking into a bowl of alphabet soup.[494] The incredible complexity of the interactions of the molecules they are researching means that they also will have far reaching effects in the body, much further than just stopping the effects of IR radiation on the skin. All these new avenues they are exploring will require extensive research to assure that the law of unintended consequences does not rear its head with this new wave of attempts at solar radiation protection.

Yes, these do sounds like novel ideas, but how do we know whether there are inherent, unforeseen problems that will appear a few years from now, just as with telling everyone to use UVB sunscreens over the past 30 years before long-term and environmental impact studies were performed. The researchers themselves state: "What is obvious is that there is a large gap in our knowledge about this response (melanocyte transformation into melanoma)."[495]

Based on past experiences of marketing chemicals prior to generational studies being performed on fish, mice or rats, which have now proven the chemicals are detrimental to life, it is best to wait until studies regarding the entire ecological impact become available before jumping on the band wagon and slathering our bodies with these newer compounds. All these are so new, we should heed one researcher's caveat: "However, it should be noted that the precise mechanism of action of topically applied actives remain to be elucidated; there is a need to fully understand their effects at both cellular and molecular levels prior to supporting their therapeutic benefits as photoprotective agents."[496]

Yet, some of the new products have already become available on the market without the extensive testing that is needed to determine whether the claims that are being made will materialize. Without aquatic and gestational studies, the products may produce undesirable results such as have been and continue to be revealed in the existing UVB and UVA sunscreen products.

Not only is it important to know the ingredients of what you place on your skin, there are also great differences in their performances based on the formulations created by the other chemicals they are mixed with, as well as the concentrations that are used.

One researcher stated:

"It has been recognized that the vehicle in which a permeant is applied to the skin has a distinctive effect on the dermal and transdermal delivery of active ingredients. The cutaneous and percutaneous absorptions can be enhanced, e.g., by an increase in thermodynamic activity, supersaturation and penetration modifiers. Furthermore, dermal and transdermal delivery can be influenced by the interactions that may occur between the vehicle and the skin on the one hand, and interactions between the active ingredient and the skin on the other hand."[497]

And another one who recently reviewed the many chemicals that are being promoted on the market for effectiveness after his review concluded:

"Although some product claims for the active ingredients used in cosmeceutical formulations are evidence-based, consumers often place their confidence in the claims made by the manufacturer. Without testing to assess the efficacy of key active ingredients in relation to overall product content, it is possible that at inadequate concentrations, any beneficial effect will become inapparent. Ensuring consistency of formulations is also an area that has been neglected and necessitates regulation."[498]

Until more is known, the safest route is to use natural strategies that are covered in Chapter 21.

As new chemicals and formulations will continually be introduced, each one needing to be researched thoroughly, this book is only the beginning of our investigations. Each new product will be fully researched, analyzed, and evaluated as to whether the claims make biochemical sense, and whether they are beneficial to put on or in our bodies. The same as for the body products, these will be covered in-depth in our ongoing *New Voice for Health Newsletter*.

Chapter 21
Protecting Yourself – Naturally

The concerns that this book covers are beginning to be voiced by the medical community. In the physicians Web-based medical information news, *Medscape*, an article about sunscreen and its use was concluded by: "However, further research is needed in many areas including the role of visible light, the risks of systemic absorption of sunscreen agents, and the role of vitamin D and sun exposure in preventing cancers and other diseases."[499]

Until these areas are clarified, it is critical for everyone to take steps that will protect the skin with natural ways that do not create more harm than good.

Australian SunSmart Program

There has been a growing concern that advice to use sunscreen may lead to longer sun exposure once "protection" is applied, which counteracts the reasons for the utilization of sunscreens. In 1982, the Australian government instituted what they called the SunSmart program, intended to reduce UV exposure, and increase use of protective clothing, hats, sunglasses, and sunscreen. Television advertisements were aimed at changing attitudes about sun tanning, and for acceptance of wearing more protective attire of "neck to knee" swimsuits for children. Due to the program, there was an increase in sun-protective behavior between 1987-2002, which correlated to a reduction in the incidence for melanoma rates in younger children. Below are their recommendations.

"However, sunscreen should not be used as the sole method of sun protection nor as a means for extending the amount of time spent in the sun. The best way for individuals to lower their risk of skin cancer is to reduce their sun exposure by combining all strategies:

> Staying out of the sun between the peak burning hours of 10 AM to 2 PM; seeking shade or bringing it (for example, a beach umbrella or tent); and wearing hats and other protective clothing, like long sleeve T-shirts and lightweight pants."

"'Building comprehensive approaches to reducing sun exposure, not just using sunscreen, are necessary to achieve our goals of reducing the burden of skin cancer.' It is not too late to cover up when in the sun and enjoy the outdoors this summer."[500]

Australian Government Requirements for Labeling Sunscreens

The Australian government's Therapeutic Goods Administration (TGS) wording regarding sunscreen labeling requires that it include the urging of avoiding prolonged sun exposure and advising to wear protective clothing. The required wording is:

"If (and only if) a therapeutic sunscreen has an SPF of 30+ and it provides broad spectrum protection, the label is permitted to include a representation to the effect that the product *'may assist in preventing some skin cancers'* or *'may reduce the risk of some skin cancers'* provided the label also highlights the need for avoidance of prolonged exposure to the sun and the importance of wearing protective clothing, hats and eyewear. Other acceptable related claims are *'can aid in the prevention of solar keratoses'* and *'can aid in the prevention of sunspots.'*"[501]

U.S. FDA 2011 Guidelines for Labeling Sunscreens

June 14, 2011, the U.S. FDA published new guidelines that outline their current recommendations. The main points in regards to labeling are listed below. A more complete listing is provided in Appendix E.

- The new regulations become effective summer 2012.
- In order to state on the label SPF 15 to a maximum of SPF 50, product has to pass a "broad spectrum" test showing that it protects against both UVA and UVB.
- If broad spectrum, claim can be made that the product protects against skin cancer and early skin aging, as well as against sunburn, if it is used as directed along with other sun protective measures:
  - o Limit time in sun between 10 AM and 2 PM.
  - o Wear protective clothing: long-sleeved shirts, pants, sunglasses, and broad-brimmed hats.
- If it does not protect against both UVA and UVB, it can only state a SPF value (cannot say broad spectrum) and only claim protection against sunburn.
- Maximum SPF of 50 allowed to be claimed as there is no sufficient data to show that products provide protection greater than SPF 50.
- Cannot claim protection unless reapplied every 2 hours.
- If water resistant: claims must state on front of label that it remains effective for 40 minutes or 80 minutes while swimming or sweating.
- If not water resistant must include a direction instructing consumers to use a water resistant sunscreen if swimming or sweating.
- Label cannot claim "waterproof" "sweatproof" or "sunblock" as this overstates their effectiveness.
- Public comment is invited before September 15, 2011.

The government agencies that are regulating sunscreens in their efforts to protect us recognize that reducing prolonged sun exposure and covering our bodies are essential even when sunscreens are utilized. Many actions can be taken that do not expose you, your family, or the planet to detrimental harm.

What You Can Do
Learn and Follow the UV Index

There is a UV Index that provides a rating of how strong the radiation of the sun will be on an hourly and daily basis world-wide. The UV radiation strength is strongest between 10 AM to 2 PM. As much as 80% of UV rays pass through clouds, so still take the same precautions on cloudy days as you would on bright, sunny days. For the index rating for your local area you can type in your city and country or state, or your ZIP code at either of the two Websites that are listed below as well as in Appendix B.

World-wide the UV index can be accessed at:

www.uvawareness.com/uv-forecast/index.php

In the U.S., the National Weather Service issues a daily forecast of UV intensity that can be accessed at:

www.epa.gov/sunwise/uvindex.html

The rating scale they both use is listed below in Table 12.

Table 12. **UV Index Rating System**

Rating	Exposure Level
<3	Low
3 to 5	Moderate
6 to 7	High
8 to 10	Very high
11+	Extreme

Source: EPA Website. Sunscreen: The Burning Facts. Available at: www.epa.gov/sunwise/doc/sunscreen.pdf.

The lower UV Index numbers would allow more sun exposure, while it is best to cover up or stay out of the sun when the index climbs to High Exposure Level and above.

Do Not Use Artificial Sun Tanning Salons

In reviewing the statistics of types of cancers among men and women and those who utilize sun tanning beds, a study published in 2007 reveals that the artificial radiation of sun tanning beds increases the risk of basal cell carcinoma, but not melanoma. However, there was not enough data to identify whether squamous cell skin cancers would be affected, but it would be best not to risk basal cell cacinomas.[502]

Do Not Use Spray-on or Airbrush Tanning Products

There are so many ingredients in the formulations that are being marketed to artificially darken the skin that it is impossible to cover all of them here. Most do contain a form of acetone, dihydroxyacetone (DHA), which even though it is considered relatively non-toxic can cause drying and irritation of the skin. Many of them only last about a week and then have to be reapplied, adding to the problem of continual drying of the skin. The most important thing in their regard to know is that the changes they create in the skin to cause the tanning can act like sunscreens, which reduces the formation of vitamin D and leads to lower body-wide vitamin D levels.[503]

Know the Medications that Increase Susceptibility to UV Rays

Certain medications increase the susceptibility to burning from the UV rays. The medications listed below increase burning with sun exposure. If you are taking any of the listed medications, do take extra care to stay protected from the sun.[504]

Always:
  Fluoroquinolones
  Sulfonamides
  Tetracyclines (especially demeclocycline)
Less frequently:
  Doxycycline
  Oxytetracycline

Rarely:
Minocycline
Thiazide diuretics
Furosemide
Amiodarone
Sulfonylureas
Acetazolamide (diamox)
Phenothiazines
Nonsteroidal anti-inflammatory drugs (naproxen, ibuprofen, aspirin)

Identify True Sun Allergies

For those who have allergic reactions to the sun, first make sure that it is not an allergy to any sunscreen lotion or body lotion that you may have applied. For some individuals an allergic reaction can occur with many of the sunscreen ingredients, particularly upon exposure to the sun. When you have determined that it is from the sun, the immune system needs to be addressed. It could be there is a toxic build up in the body or heavy metal poisoning of the liver. To rule this out, seek a doctor's help for toxin removal.

Action Steps to Take

Rather than use chemicals, there are many steps you can take to protect yourself from UV rays.

- Seek shade, cover up, and avoid the sun between 10 AM and 2 PM.
- Be extra careful when the UV Index is high.
- Be extra careful near water, snow, and sand as they reflect and intensify the radiation.
- Do not use sun tanning products or tanning beds.

Know What You Put on Your Body and into Your Body

The biochemistry of the body is extremely complicated, to say the least. Know what you are putting on your skin, the largest organ of your body, as it readily and rapidly absorbs what is put on it. Read every label for body lotions, cosmetics, clothing, and swimwear. When they state a rating for UV protection, find out what chemicals have been used for the protection, as sun filtering chemicals including TiO_2 are appearing in many products. One of the authors of the 2009 UCLA *Cancer Research* article on TiO_2 nanoparticles stated:

"The manufacture of TiO_2 nanoparticles is a huge industry," Dr. Schiestl said, "with production at about 2 million tons per year. In addition to paint, cosmetics, sunscreen and vitamins, the nanoparticles can be found in toothpaste, food colorants, nutritional supplements and hundreds of other personal care products." He voiced his concern over these products due to his UCLA study that lead to the conclusions: "In the past, these TiO_2 nanoparticles have been considered non-toxic in that they do not incite a chemical reaction. Instead, it is surface interactions that the nanoparticles have within their environment – in this case inside a mouse – that is causing the genetic damage, Schiestl said. They wander throughout the body causing oxidative stress, which can lead to cell death."[505]

Even when the product is not advertised that it is for sun protection, still read the labels. Read all the over-the-counter medications as TiO_2 nanoparticles are added to some (e.g., Benadryl). Also read every label in natural health food stores. Pure and natural soaps with only a handful of ingredients can still contain TiO_2, which will be in the nanoparticle form even though they are not required to include that information on the label.

Products containing TiO_2 nanoparticles are being promoted for everything. It is "Buyer Beware". Websites have cropped up promoting them as safe and even that they are for a greener planet. Everything from self-cleaning toilets, deodorant bars, air purifiers, and water filters to paint have had these minute particles added. They are not safe or good for the planet; they are not only hazardous to your health, they are hazardous to the health of the planet. Check the labels on everything you buy and refuse to buy products that incorporate either TiO_2 or ZnO nanoparticles. When there is no market for their products, the manufacturers will stop utilizing them.

Throw Sunscreen Chemicals in Hazardous Waste Stations

Read the labels of all of your skin care products. Throw out all of those that include any of the chemicals listed in Appendix C. Make sure to dispose of them in your community's hazardous waste area and not into the main garbage, as they need to be removed from the environment.

Select Sun Shielding Clothes

Select tightly woven fabrics of darker colors. To determine whether clothing can block the sun's rays, it can be held up to the light to determine whether light is coming through it or not. A good material for blocking the rays is tightly knit denim.

Sun protective behavior can become part of our lives again. Umbrellas can be used for shade. An umbrella with tightly women fabric would provide protection, and is a better choice for your health than those that are being manufactured with TiO_2 nanoparticles. Women can start making the wearing of gloves fashionable again, just like it was only 50 short years ago. Swimming attire that covers more of the body, especially for our children and babies like the campaign on Australian television, can also become the new "normal" for sensible sun behavior.

Reduce the Amount of Time Spent in the Sun

There are common sense answers for everything, including our sunbathing behavior. There needs to be a balance to everything. Sunscreens have created a false sense of security. We were not designed to stay in the sun as long as sunscreens have allowed us to by blocking out our red warning light – a sunburn. By doing so, we have artificially stopped a natural protection process.

Avoid Commercial Chemical and Physical Sunscreens

At the time of this writing, I have not discovered any products that claim sunscreen protection that do not incorporate at least one of the chemicals, or the physical blockers that have been identified in this book as being harmful for humans as well as for the planet. They are products that were put on the market without adequate testing. We cannot chemically treat ourselves without disrupting the body's ecosystem, and the environmental ecosystem of the planet's lakes, rivers, and oceans.

Adopt Antioxidants

Adopt antioxidants in your diet and for your skin as a way of life. They not only will protect your skin, they will generate health throughout your body. They are especially essential for our survival in today's toxic filled world.

Call to Action

The perceptions of the sun's potential for cancerous changes and creating damage that leads to skin aging have been utilized as the impetus to elicit cooperation of protecting the skin with sunscreen preparations. The call to action today needs to be turned toward protecting life on the planet as we know it. For the health of our bodies and developing babies, and for survival of both fresh and salt water fish, we humans have to stop using all these sunscreen preparations and switch to nature's sunscreens — the antioxidants. Utilize clothing that covers our bodies and stay out of the sun as our ancestors used to before sunscreens allowed us to circumvent our warning sunburn and encouraged us to stay in the sun much longer than is healthy for our skin.[506]

These concerns and proof of harm to life have shown up throughout the entire lifetime of sun filtering products being offered to consumers. Yet warning labels have not been required and the manufacturers have not volunteered to pull them off the market in concern of the safety of human beings and preservation of the aquatic and marine life on the planet. However, this lack of response threatens our very existence on the planet, because if our oceans die off — humankind will not be far behind. It is imperative that we only use products that protect our health, our unborn children's brains and natural sexual development, and preserve the incredible array of life in the ocean that feeds us and sustains us, and provides such a great playground for our enjoyment.

New Voice for Health Newsletter

Ongoing Research

We will be continually researching and finding the best make-ups, body lotions, sunning products, and antioxidants so that you can truly enjoy your time in the sun without worrying about cancerous changes or photoaging. As there are constantly new ideas and products emerging on the sunscreen market, the *New Voice for Health Newsletter* will provide the same critical examination and in-depth analysis of the studies and medical advice that you have seen throughout this book. Our goal is for you to have the clarity you need to make informed decisions as to whether utilizing the latest discovery is the right course of action for you and your family. It will provide information regarding the most current knowledge regarding:

Vitamin D:
 How much time in the sun?
 How much to take as a supplement?
 Optimal blood levels?

Products that are safe:
 Make up.
 Body lotions.
 Sunning lotions.

Antioxidants:
 Which are best?
 How to use?

Clearing sunscreen chemicals:
From your body.
Best and safest methods?

At only $39 per year, it will be the best investment you will ever make as we will be conducting the 100s of hours of research it takes to determine if a new product is actually safe, sensible, and whether it is truly beneficial for your body, your skin, your children, and protects our environment.

Sign up for the newsletter at:

www.sunscreensbiohazard.com/newsletter.htm

Or mail your name and address to:

New Voice for Health
P.O. Box 14133
Irvine, CA 92623

We would love to stay in touch and keep you on top of the latest information available.

May you live a healthy and productive life,

♥ *Elizabeth*

Appendix A
Antioxidant Sources

ORAC Antioxidant Values List and Website Link.

An updated list of ORAC values is available at:

www.ars.usda.gov/SP2UserFiles/Place/12354500/Data/ORAC/
ORAC_R2.pdf

Antioxidant Food and Supplement Sources

List in Alphabetical Order

Alfalfa sprouts		
Alpha lipoic acid		
Apples	2,500	ORAC value
Artichokes	9,400	
Asparagus	2,150	
Avocado	1,370	
Baking chocolate, unsweetened	50,000	
Beef		
Black tea	1,100	
Blackberries	4,000	
Blueberries, raw wild	10,000	
Bok choy		
Bright colored fruits and vegetables		
Broccoli, boiled	2,100	
raw	1,350	
Brown rice		

Brussels sprouts
Cabbage
Cabbage, green   500
Cabbage, red   2,400
Cantaloupe   300
Capers
Carrots   700
Cauliflower
Cauliflower sprouts
Cheese
Chicken livers
Cocoa (mixed powder)   485
Coffee
Crab
Crawfish
Cruciferous vegetables
Crustaceans
Dairy: cheese (cottage and ricotta),
      eggs, yogurt, milk
Eggplant   900
Eggs
Elderberries   14,700
Fish oil
Flavonoids
Garlic   5,500
Genistein (soybeans)
Goji berry juice
Grains: oats, wheat germ, granola
Grapefruit   1,600
Green leafy vegetables
Green tea   1,300
Kale

King oyster mushrooms	
Krill	
Lobster	
Maitake mushrooms	700
Microalgae	
Milk	
Milk thistle	
N–acetylcysteine	
Oats	
Olive oil	
Omega-3 fatty acids	
Onions, raw	900
Oranges, raw	2,000
Oyster mushrooms	700
Peach	1,900
Peanuts, raw	3,200
Pineapples	600
Plums	8,000
Pomegranates	4,500
Pork	
Potatoes	1,600
Poultry	
Rainbow trout	
Raspberries, raw	5,100
Red cabbage, raw	2,500
Red colored fish and shellfish	
Red grapes	1,800
Red peppers	800
Rice bran	24,300
Rosemary dried	165,000
Salmon	
SAMe	

Selenium (sources: Brazil nuts, meats, sea foods).
Shiitake mushrooms, dried   800
Shrimp
Spinach, raw   1,500
Squash, zucchini   400
Strawberries   4,300
Turnips
Vitamin Bs: B12, B6, B2
   (riboflavin), and folate
Vitamin C
Vitamin E
Watercress
Watermelon   100
Wheat germ
White tea   300
Whole wheat
Yeast

Spices:

Basil, dried	61,000	ORAC value
Basil, fresh	4,800	
Chili powder	24,000	
Cinnamon, ground	130,000	
Cloves, ground	290,000	
Cumin seed	50,000	
Curry powder	49,000	
Ginger, ground	39,000	
Marjoram, fresh	27,000	
Mustard seeds	29,000	
Nutmeg, ground	70,000	
Oregano, dried	175,000	
Oregano, fresh	14,000	

Parsley, dried	74,000
Pepper black	34,000
Rosemary, dried	165,000
Sage, ground	120,000
Szechwan pepper, dried	118,000
Tarragon, fresh	16,000
Thyme, dried	157,000
Thyme, fresh	27,000
Turmeric, ground	127,000
Vanilla beans	122,000

Polyphenols and Their Food Sources

The broad categories of polyphenols are the flavonols, isoflavones, anthocyanins, flavanols, and flavanones. Favones are found in sweet red peppers and celery. Genistein is an isoflavone found in soy, but it is estrogenic and not recommended when building up antioxidant activity as a sunscreen. Flavanones are in citrus fruits, with specific ones found in oranges. Anthocyanidins are in the red fruits such as cherries, plums, strawberries, raspberries, blackberries, grapes, red currants and black currants. The flavonol quercetin is found in yellow and red, but not white onions, as well as tea. Flavanols are the catechins found in tea, red wine, and chocolate; the proanthocyanidin is in apple peels, pears, grapes red wine, tea, and chocolate. Ferulic acids are found under phenolic acids, with wheat bran being one of the richest sources. Caffeic acid is another phenolic acid that is found in coffee. Gallic acid is in mangos. Lignans are enterodiols that are found in flax seed and flax seed oil. The best known stilbene is resveratrol.[507]

Food Sources for Specific Antioxidants
Carotenoid sources:

Fresh thyme, fresh	27,500	ORAC value
Cilantro	5,100	
Sweet potatoes baked	2,100	
Carrots	700	
Winter squash	400	

Leafy greens:
  Kale
  Spinach
  Turnip greens
  Collard greens

Flavonoid sources:

Plants, especially fruits

Blueberries	10,000
Artichokes	9,400
Soybeans	5,400
Raspberries raw	5,100
Raspberry seed oil [provides a sunscreen protection of SPF 28-50]	
Strawberries	4,300
Cabbage red, boiled	3,100
raw	2,500
Apples (quercetin)	2,500
Beans, black	2,300
Parsley, raw	1,300
Apricots raw	1,100
Beans, pinto	900
Cabbage green, boiled	900
raw	500
Onions, raw	900

Tomatoes	400
Citrus fruits	

Tea [about 25% flavonoids whether
green or black tea]:

Green tea	1,300
Black tea	1,100
White tea	300

Polyphenol sources:

Berries

Acai	103,000
Blueberries, wild	10,000
Blueberries	5,000
Blackberries	5,900
Raspberries	5,100
Strawberries	4,300
Prunes, dried	8,100
Pomegranates, raw	4,500
Cherries raw sweet	3,800
Cherry-black juice	2,400
Cabbage red, boiled	3,200
raw	2,500
Pomegranate juice	2,700
Apples	2,500
Broccoli, boiled	2,200
raw	1,500
Beet greens, raw	2,000
Oranges	2,000
Red grapes, raw	1,800
Grapefruits, raw	1,600
Cranberry juice	1,500

Spinach	1,500
Tea	
Green	1,300
Black	1,100
White	300
Onions, raw	900
Celery, raw	600
Peas green, frozen	600
Olive oil	400
Cantaloupe	300
Beans	
Buckwheat	
Nuts	
Oats	
Olives	
Sesame seeds	
Soybeans	

Selenium sources:
Barley
Oats

Vitamin C sources:

Blueberries, wild	10,000
Blueberries	5,000
Artichokes	9,400
Pomegranates	4,000
Broccoli, raw	3,000
Cabbage red, boiled	3,000
Pomegranate juice	2,700
Oranges	2,000
Avocados	1,900

Peaches	1,900
Onions red, raw	1,500
Romaine lettuce	1,000
Cabbage green, boiled	900
Onions white, raw	900
Red peppers	800
Sweet potatoes	800
Tomatoes	400
Brussels sprouts	
Kale	
Swiss chard	
Watercress	

Vitamin E sources:

Grains – wheat, rice, barley, oats	
Almonds	4,500
Spinach	1,500
Brazil nuts	1,400
Tomatoes	400
Olives	
Sunflower seeds	
Oils – sunflower, palm, and olive oil	400

Appendix B
UV Index Rating System

The index rating for your local area is available when you type in your city and country or state, or your ZIP code.

World-wide the UV index can be accessed at:

www.uvawareness.com/uv-forecast/index.php

In the U.S., the National Weather Service issues a daily forecast of UV intensity that can be accessed at:

www.epa.gov/sunwise/uvindex.html

Table 12. **UV Index Rating System**

Rating	Exposure Level
<3	Low
3 to 5	Moderate
6 to 7	High
8 to 10	Very high
11+	Extreme

Appendix C
Sunscreen Chemicals

The chemicals are listed in several ways, starting with alphabetical order first. Some have many names so could appear elsewhere in the list utilizing a different name first in the alphabetical order. This is designed so you can rapidly identify the chemicals in ingredient lists of products that you are considering buying.

Attempts were made to make these lists as complete as possible, however there are many more names for these chemicals as well as new ones being added continually.

Alphabetical Listing
(Those starting with numbers can be found at the bottom of the lists.)

Advastab 45 (BP3)
Amiloxate (Neo Heliopan E1000)
Anuvex (BP3)
Avobenzone
Bemotrizinol (Tinosorb S)
Benzoic acid, 2-[4-(diethylamino)-2- hydroxybenzoyl]-hexyl ester
    (Uvinul A Plus)
Benzophenone 5 (BP5)
Benzophenone-1 (BP1)
Benzophenone-2 (BP2)
Benzophenone-2 bis(2,4-dihydroxyphenyl) methanone (BP2)
Benzophenone-3 (BP3)
Benzophenone-4 (BP4)
Bis-ethylhexyloxyphenol methoxyphenyl triazine (Tinosorb S)

Bisoctrizol (Tinosorb M)
BMDBM (Avobenzone)
BP1
BP2
BP3
BP4
BP5
BP6
BP8
Butyl methoxy dibenzoylmethane (Avobenzone)
Camphor benzalkonium methosulfate N,N,N-trimethyl-4-(oxoborn-3-ylidenemethyl) anilinium methyl sulfate (BP8)
Chimassorb 90 (BP3)
Cinoxate
Cyasorb UV 9 (BP3)
Diethylamino hydroxybenzoyl hexyl benzoate (Uvinul A Plus)
Dioxybenzone (BP9)
Dioxybenzone benzophenone 8 (BP8)
Disodium phenyl dibenzimidazole tetrasulfonate (Neo Heliopn)
DPDT (Neo Heliopn)
Drometrizole trisiloxane (Mexoryl XL)
Drometrizole trisiloxane phenol
Ecamsule
EHT (Uvinul T 150)
EMC (Octinoxate)
Enzacamene (4-MBC)
Escalol 507 (OD-PABA)
Escalol 557 (Octinoxate)
Escalol 567 (BP3)
Escalol 577 (BP4)
Escalol 587 (Octisalate)
Ethoxylated ethyl-4-aminobenzoic acid (PEG25 PABA)

Ethylhexyl triazone (Uvinul T 150)
Ethylmethoxycinnamate (Octinoxate)
Eusolex 4360 (BP3)
Eusolex 6300 (4-MBC)
Eusolex 9020 (Avobenzone)
Eusolex OCR (Octocrylene)
HMS
Homomethyl salicylate (HMS)
Homosalate (HMS)
IMC (Neo Heliopan E1000)
Isoamyl methoxycinnamateIsopentenyl-4-methoxycinnamate (Neo
    Heliopan E1000)
Isoamyl p-methoxycinnamate (Neo Heliopan E1000)
Isopropylbenzyl salicylate
MBC (4-MBC)
Menthyl anthranilate
Methyl 2-aminobenzoate
Methylene bis-benzotriazolyl tetramethylbutyl phenol (Tinosorb M)
Mexoryl SX (Ecamsule)
Mexoryl XL
MOB (BP3)
Neo Heliopan
Neo Heliopan E1000
Octinoxate
Octisalate
Octocrylene
Octyl dimethyl-PABA (OD-PABA)
Octyl methoxycinnamate (Octinoxate)
Octyl salicylate (Octisalate)
Octyl triazone (Uvinul T 150)
Octyl triazone 2,4,6-trianalino-(p-carbo-2'-ethylhexyl-1'oxy)1,3,5-
    triazine

OD-PABA
σ-PABA (OD-PABA)
OMC (Octinoxate)
Ongrostab HMB (BP3)
Oxybenzone (BP3)
Oxybenzophenone (BP3)
PABA
Padimate O (OD-PABA)
p-aminobenzoic acid (PABA)
Parsol 1789 (Avobenzone)
Parsol 5000 (4-MBC)
Parsol MCX (Octinoxate)
Parsol SLX
PEG-25 PABA
Phenylbenzimidazole sulfonic acid
Polysilicone-15 (Parsol SLX)
Spectra-Sorb UV-9 (BP3)
Sulisobenzone (BP4)
Sulisobenzone sodium (BP5)
Sunscreen UV 15 (BP3)
Syntase 62 (BP3)
Terephthalylidene dicamphor sulfonic acid (Ecamsule)
Tinosorb M
Tinosorb S
Titanium dioxide
Triethanolamine salicylate
UF 3 (BP3)
Uvinul 9 (BP3)
Uvinul A Plus
Uvinul M-40 (BP3)
Uvinul N 539 T
Uvinul P 25 (PEG-25 PABA)

Uvinul T 150
Uvistat 24 (BP3)
Zinc oxide (ZnO)
1-(4-methoxyphenyl)-3-(4-tert-butyl phenyl)propane-1,3-dione
   (Avobenzone)
2-(2H-benzotriazol-2-yl)-4- methyl-6[2-methyl-2,2'-dihydroxy-4,4'-
   dimethoxybenzophenone (BP6)
2-benzoyl-5-methoxyphenol (BP3)
2-cyano-3,3diphenyl acrylic acid (Octocrylene)
2-ethylhexyl 4-dimethylaminobenzoate (OD-PABA)
2-ethylhexyl salicylate (Octisalate)
2-ethylhexylester (Octocrylene)
2-ethylhexyl-paramethoxycinnamate (Octinoxate)
2-hydroxy-4-methoxybenzophenone (HMB) (BP3)
2-Hydroxy-4-methoxybenzophenone-5-sulfonic acid (BP4)
2-Hydroxy-4-methoxyphenyl-phenylmethanone (BP3)
3-[1,3,3,3- tetramethyl-1-(trimethylsilyl)oxy]disiloxanyl]propy l
   3-benzoyl-4-hydroxy-6-methoxybenzenesulfonic acid (BP4)
3-BC
4,4'-dihydroxybenzophenone (4DHB)
4-isopropylbenzyl salicylate
4-hydroxy benzophenone (4HB)
4-MBC
4-methylbenzylidene camphor (4-MBC)

Listing by Country Approval

The sunscreen chemicals are listed with their most common name first, with the names they are also know as below them. If at first you do not see the name, keep looking in the second tier of names.

U.S. FDA Approved

Avobenzone – also known by the names:
BMDBM
Butyl methoxy dibenzoylmethane
Escalol 517
Eusolex 9020
Parsol 1789
1-(4-methoxyphenyl)-3-(4-tert-butyl phenyl)propane-1,3-dione
4-tert-butyl-4-methoxydibenzoyl-methane
BP3 – also known by the names:
Advastab 45
Anuvex
Benzophenone-3
Chimassorb 90
Cyasorb UV 9
Escalol 567
Escalol 567
Eusolex 4360
MOB
Ongrostab HMB
Oxybenzone
Oxybenzophenone
Spectra-Sorb UV-9
Sunscreen UV 15
Syntase 62
UF 3

Uvinul 9
Uvinul M-40
Uvistat 24
2-benzoyl-5-methoxyphenol
2-hydroxy-4-methoxybenzophenone (HMB)
2-hydroxy-4-methoxyphenyl-phenylmethanone
BP4 – also known by the names:
    Benzophenone-4
    Escalol 577
    Sulisobenzone
    Uvinul MS 40
    2-hydroxy-4-methoxybenzophenone-5-sulfonic acid
    3-benzoyl-4-hydroxy-6-methoxybenzenesulfonic acid
BP8 – also known by the name:
    Dioxybenzone benzophenone 8
Cinoxate
Ecamsule: as Anthelios
Homosalate – also known by the names:
    HMS
    Homomethyl salicylate
Menthyl anthranilate – also known by the names:
    MA
    Meradimate
    Methyl-2-aminobenzoate
Octinoxate – also known by the names:
    EHMC
    EMC
    Escalol 557
    Ethylmethoxycinnamate
    Eusolex 2292
    Octyl methoxycinnamate
    OMC

Parsol MCX
Uvinul MC80
2-EHMC
2-ethylhexyl-paramethoxycinnamate
Octocrylene – also known by the names:
    Eusolex OCR
    Uvinul N 539 T
    2-cyano-3,3diphenyl acrylic acid
    2-ethylhexylester
Octyl salicylate – also known by the names:
    Escalol 587
    Octisalate
    2-ethylhexyl salicylate
PABA – also known by the names:
    p-aminobenzoic acid
    4-aminobenzoic acid
Padimate O – also known by the names:
    Escalol 507
    Octyl dimethyl-PABA
    OD-PABA
    σ-PABA
    2-ethylhexyl 4-dimethylaminobenzoate
PBSA – also known by the names:
    Ensulizole
    Eusolex 232
    Parsol HS
    Phenylbenzimidazole 5-sulfonic acid
Titanium dioxide
Trolamine salicylate
Zinc oxide (ZnO)

European Union Approved

Avobenzone – also known by the names:
    BMDBM
    Butyl methoxy dibenzoylmethane
    Escalol 517
    Eusolex 9020
    Parsol 1789
    1-(4-methoxyphenyl)-3-(4-tert-butyl phenyl)propane-1,3-dione
BP3 – also known by the names:
    Benzophenone-3
    Escalol 567
    Eusolex 4360
    Oxybenzone
BP4 – also known by the names:
    Benzophenone-4
    Escalol 577
    Sulisobenzone
    Uvinul MS 40
    2-hydroxy-4-methoxybenzophenone-5-sulfonic acid
    3-benzoyl-4-hydroxy-6-methoxybenzenesulfonic acid
Ecamsule – also known by the names:
    Mexoryl SX
    Terephthalylidene dicamphor sulfonic acid
Homosalate – also known by the names:
    HMS
    Homomethyl salicylate
Mexoryl XL – also known by the name:
    Drometrizole trisiloxane
Neo Heliopan E1000 – also known by the names:
    Amiloxate
    IMC
    Isoamyl methoxycinnamateIsopentenyl-4-methoxycinnamate
    Isoamyl p-methoxycinnamate

Octinoxate – also known by the names:
    EHMC
    EMC
    Escalol 557
    Ethylmethoxycinnamate
    Eusolex 2292
    Octyl methoxycinnamate
    OMC
    Parsol MCX
    Uvinul MC80
    2-EHMC
    2-ethylhexyl-paramethoxycinnamate
Octocrylene – also known by the names:
    Eusolex OCR
    Uvinul N 539 T
    2-cyano-3,3diphenyl acrylic acid
    2-ethylhexylester
Octyl salicylate – also known by the names:
    Escalol 587
    Octisalate
    2-ethylhexyl salicylate
PABA – also known by the names:
    p-aminobenzoic acid
    4-aminobenzoic acid
Padimate O – also known by the names:
    Escalol 507
    Octyl dimethyl-PABA
    OD-PABA
    σ-PABA
    2-ethylhexyl 4-dimethylaminobenzoate
Parsol SLX – also known by the names:
    Dimethico-diethylbenzalmalonate
    Polysilicone-15

PBSA – also known by the names:
    Ensulizole
    Eusolex 232
    Parsol HS
    Phenylbenzimidazole 5-sulfonic acid
Tinosorb M – also known by the names:
    Bisoctrizol
    MBBT
    Methylene bis-benzotriazolyl tetramethylbutyl phenol
Tinosorb S – also known by the names:
    Bemotrizinol
    BEMT
    Bis-ethylhexyloxyphenol methoxyphenyl triazine
Titanium dioxide
Uvasorb HEB – also known by the names:
    DBT
    Diethylhexyl butamido triazone
    Iscotrizinol
Uvinul A Plus – also known by the name:
    Diethylamino hydroxybenzoyl hexyl benzoate
Uvinul T 150 – also known by the names:
    EHT
    Ethylhexyl triazone
    Octyl triazone
Zinc oxide (ZnO)
4-MBC – also known by the names:
    Enzacamene
    Eusolex 6300
    MBC
    Parsol 5000
    4-methylbenzylidene camphor. (EU Scientific Committee on
        Consumer Products Report approving 4-MBC.)[508]
        [This European Union report is available at: http://ec.europa.eu/
        health/ph_risk/committees/04_sccp/docs/sccp_o_141.pdf.]

Australia Approved

Avobenzone – also known by the names:

BMDBM

Butyl methoxy dibenzoylmethane

Escalol 517

Eusolex 9020

Parsol 1789

1-(4-methoxyphenyl)-3-(4-tert-butyl phenyl)propane-1,3-dione

BP2 – also known by the names:

Benzophenone-2

Benzophenone-2 bis(2,4-dihydroxyphenyl) methanone (under review)

BP3 – also known by the names:

Benzophenone-3

Escalol 567

Eusolex 4360

Oxybenzone

BP4 – also known by the names:

Benzophenone-4

Escalol 577

Sulisobenzone

Uvinul MS 40

2-hydroxy-4-methoxybenzophenone-5-sulfonic acid

3-benzoyl-4-hydroxy-6-methoxybenzenesulfonic acid

BP5 – also known by the names:

Benzophenone 5

Sulisobenzone sodium

BP6 – also known by the name:

2,2'-dihydroxy-4,4'-dimethoxybenzophenone

BP8 – also known by the name:

Dioxybenzone benzophenone 8

Camphor benzalkonium methosulfate, N,N,N-Trimethyl-4-
(oxoborn-3-ylidenemethyl) anilinium methyl sulfate

Cinoxate
Drometrizole trisiloxane phenol, 2-(2H-benzotriazol-2-yl)-4- methyl-
6[2-methyl-3-[1,3,3,3- tetramethyl-1- (trimethylsilyl)oxy]
disiloxanyl]propy l
Ecamsule – also known by the names:
  Mexoryl SX
  Terephthalylidene dicamphor sulfonic acid
Homosalate – also known by the names:
  HMS
  Homomethyl salicylate
Isopropylbenzyl salicylate – also known by the name:
  4-isopropylbenzyl salicylate (under review)
Menthyl anthranilate – also known by the names:
  MA
  Meradimate
  Methyl 2-aminobenzoate
Mexoryl XL – also known by the name:
  Drometrizole trisiloxane
Neo Heliopan – also known by the name:
  Disodium phenyl dibenzimidazole tetrasulfonate
Neo Heliopan E1000 – also known by the names:
  Amiloxate
  IMC
  Isoamyl methoxycinnamateIsopentenyl-4-methoxycinnamate
  Isoamyl p-methoxycinnamate
Octinoxate – also known by the names:
  EHMC
  EMC
  Escalol 557
  Ethylmethoxycinnamate
  Eusolex 2292
  Octyl methoxycinnamate

OMC
Parsol MCX
Uvinul MC80
2-EHMC
2-ethylhexyl-paramethoxycinnamate
Octocrylene – also known by the names:
Eusolex OCR
Uvinul N 539 T
2-cyano-3,3diphenyl acrylic acid
2-ethylhexylester
Octyl salicylate – also known by the names:
Escalol 587
Octisalate
2-ethylhexyl salicylate
Octyl triazone 2,4,6-trianalino-(p-carbo-2'-ethylhexyl-1'oxy)1,3,5-
triazine
PABA – also known by the names:
p-aminobenzoic acid (under review)
4-aminobenzoic acid
Padimate O – also known by the names:
Escalol 507
Octyl dimethyl-PABA
OD-PABA
σ-PABA
2-ethylhexyl 4-dimethylaminobenzoate
Parsol SLX – also known by the names:
Polysilicone-15
Dimethicodiethylbenzalmalonate
PBSA – also known by the names:
Ensulizole
Eusolex 232
Parsol HS
Phenylbenzimidazole 5-sulfonic acid

PEG-25 PABA – also known by the names:
    Ethoxylated ethyl-4-aminobenzoic acid PEG25 PABA
    Uvinul P 25
Tinosorb M – also known by the names:
    Bisoctrizol
    Methylene bis-benzotriazolyl tetramethylbutyl phenol
Tinosorb S – also known by the names:
    Bemotrizinol
    BEMT
    Bis-ethylhexyloxyphenol methoxyphenyl triazine
Titanium dioxide
Triethanolamine salicylate
Uvinul A Plus – also known by the names:
    Benzoic acid, 2-[4-(diethylamino)-2- hydroxybenzoyl]-hexyl
        ester
    Diethylamino hydroxybenzoyl hexyl benzoate
Uvinul T 150 – also known by the names:
    EHT
    Ethylhexyl triazone
    Octyl triazone
Zinc oxide (ZnO)
4-MBC – also known by the names:
    Enzacamene
    Eusolex 6300
    MBC
    Parsol 5000
    4-methylbenzylidene camphor

Japan Approved

Avobenzone – also known by the names:

BMDBM

Butyl methoxy dibenzoylmethane

Escalol 517

Eusolex 9020

Parsol 1789

1-(4-methoxyphenyl)-3-(4-tert-butyl phenyl)propane-1,3-dione

BP3 – also known by the names:

Benzophenone-3

Escalol 567

Eusolex 4360

Oxybenzone

BP4 – also known by the names:

Benzophenone-4

Escalol 577

Sulisobenzone

Uvinul MS 40

2-hydroxy-4-methoxybenzophenone-5-sulfonic acid

3-benzoyl-4-hydroxy-6-methoxybenzenesulfonic acid

BP9 – also known by the names:

CAS 3121-60-6

Sodium dihydroxy dimethoxy disulfobenzophenone

Uvinul DS 49

Homosalate – also known by the names:

HMS

Homomethyl salicylate

Octinoxate – also known by the names:

EHMC

EMC

Escalol 557

Ethylmethoxycinnamate

Eusolex 2292
Octyl methoxycinnamate
OMC
Parsol MCX
Uvinul MC80
2-EHMC
2-ethylhexyl-paramethoxycinnamate
Octocrylene – also known by the names:
    Eusolex OCR
    Uvinul N 539 T
    2-cyano-3,3diphenyl acrylic acid
    2-ethylhexylester
Octyl salicylate (salicylate) – also known by the names:
    Escalol 587
    Octisalate
    2-ethylhexyl salicylate
Padimate O – also known by the names:
    Escalol 507
    OD-PABA
    Octyl dimethyl-PABA
    σ-PABA
    2-ethylhexyl 4-dimethylaminobenzoate
Parsol SLX – also known by the names:
    Polysilicone-15
    Dimethicodiethylbenzalmalonate
PBSA – also known by the names:
    Ensulizole
    Eusolex 232
    Parsol HS
    Phenylbenzimidazole 5-sulfonic acid
Tinosorb M – also known by the names:
    Bisoctrizol
    Methylene bis-benzotriazolyl tetramethylbutyl phenol

Tinosorb S – also known by the names:
Bemotrizinol
BEMT
Bis-ethylhexyloxyphenol methoxyphenyl triazine
Titanium dioxide
Uvasorb HEB – also known by the names:
DBT
Diethylhexyl butamido triazone
Iscotrizinol
Uvinul A Plus – also known by the name:
Diethylamino hydroxybenzoyl hexyl benzoate
Zinc oxide (ZnO)

Listing by Solar Wavelengths Filtered
UVA
Avobenzone – also known by the names:
BMDBM
Butyl methoxy dibenzoylmethane
Escalol 517
Eusolex 9020
Parsol 1789
1-(4-methoxyphenyl)-3-(4-tert-butyl phenyl)propane-1,3-dione
Methyl anthranilate – also known by the names:
MA
Meradimate
Methyl 2-aminobenzoate
Mexoryl SX – also known by the name:
Ecamsule
Neo Heliopan AP – also known by the name:
Bisdisulizole disodium
Uvinul A Plus – also known by the name:
Diethylamino hydroxybenzoyl hexyl benzoate

UVB

Camphors:

3-BC

4-MBC – also known by the names:

Enzacamene

Eusolex 6300

MBC

Parsol 5000

4-methylbenzylidene camphor

Cinnamates – also known by the names:

Cinoxate

EHMC

EMC

Escalol 557

Ethylmethoxycinnamate

Eusolex 2292

Octinoxate

Octyl methoxycinnamate

OMC

Parsol MCX

Uvinul MC80

2-EHMC

2-ethylhexyl-paramethoxycinnamate

PABA – also known by the names:

p-aminobenzoic acid

4-aminobenzoic acid

Padimate O – also known by the names:

Escalol 507

Octyl dimethyl-PABA

OD-PABA

σ-PABA

2-ethylhexyl 4-dimethylaminobenzoate

Parsol SLX – also known by the names:
Dimethicodiethylbenzalmalonate
Polysilicone-15
Salicylates
Homosalate (HMS)
Octyl salicylate, (octisalate), (OS) – also known by the names:
Escalol 587
Ethylhexyl salicylate
Uvinul T 150 – also known by the names:
EHT
Ethylhexyl triazone
Octyl triazone

UVA + UVB
All benzophenones 1-12 (see under other names listed above.)
Benzophenone 1
Benzophenone 2
Benzophenone 3 oxybenzone
Benzophenone 4 sulisobenzone
Benzophenone 5 sulisobenzone sodium
Benzophenone 6
Benzophenone 7
Benzophenone 8 dioxybenzone
Benzophenone 9
Benzophenone 10
Benzophenone 11
Benzophenone 12
Mexoryl XL – also known by the name:
Drometrizole trisiloxane

Octocrylene – also known by the names:
    Eusolex OCR
    Uvinul N 539 T
    2-cyano-3,3diphenyl acrylic acid
    2-ethylhexylester
PBSA – also known by the names:
    Ensulizole
    Eusolex 232
    Parsol HS
    Phenylbenzimidazole 5-sulfonic acid
Tinosorb M – also known by the names:
    Bisoctrizole
    Chemical/physical 200nm hybrid with titanium dioxide/zinc oxide
Tinosorb S – also known by the names:
    Bemotrizinol
    BEMT
    Bis-ethylhexyloxyphenol methoxyphenyl triazine
Titanium dioxide (TiO_2)
Uvasorb HEB – also known by the names:
    DBT
    Diethylhexyl butamido triazone
    Iscotrizinol
Zinc oxide (ZnO)

Appendix D
Toxic Ingredients Searches

To determine whether the products you are using everyday, or want to purchase, have toxic ingredients see the National Institute of Health Website at:

http://householdproducts.nlm.nih.gov/

Appendix E
FDA Guidelines
Published June 14, 2011

Questions and Answers: FDA announces new requirements for over-the-counter (OTC) sunscreen products marketed in the U.S.

On June 14, 2011 the U.S. Food and Drug Administration (FDA) announced new requirements for sunscreens currently sold over-the-counter (OTC) (i.e. non-prescription). These requirements support the Agency's ongoing efforts to ensure that sunscreens meet modern-day standards for safety and effectiveness. The new requirements, as well as several proposed changes for future rules, are outlined in four regulatory documents that include a Final Rule, a Proposed Rule, an Advance Notice of Proposed Rulemaking, and a Draft Guidance for Industry.

The following questions and answers provide a brief overview of the recent regulatory actions and highlight the most important information for consumers to know when buying and using sunscreen products.

Questions

Q1. Why is FDA making changes to how sunscreens are marketed in the United States?

Q2. When will these changes take effect?

Q3. What do consumers need to know when buying and using sunscreens?

Q4. What are the main points of the new Final Rule?

Q5. What does the Proposed Rule address?

Q6. What is the purpose of the Advance Notice of Proposed Rulemaking (ANPR)?

Q7. Why is the Advance Notice of Proposed Rulemaking (ANPR) requesting additional data on sunscreen products in the form of sprays?

Q8. What is included in the Draft Guidance for Industry?

Q9. Why isn't FDA finalizing all the proposed sunscreen changes under one rule?

Q10. Where can I find more information on these various regulatory actions?

Questions and Answers

Q1. Why is FDA making changes to how sunscreens are marketed in the United States?

A. FDA is making changes to how sunscreens are marketed in the United States as part of the Agency's ongoing efforts to ensure that sunscreens meet modern-day standards for safety and effectiveness and help consumers have the information they need so they can choose the right sun protection for themselves and their families. Prior rules on sunscreens dealt almost exclusively with protection against only ultraviolet B (UVB) radiation from the sun, and did not address skin cancer and early skin aging caused by ultraviolet A (UVA) rays. After reviewing the latest science, FDA determined that sufficient data are available to establish a standard broad spectrum test procedure that measures UVA radiation protection in relation to the amount of UVB radiation protection. This designation will give consumers better information on which sunscreen products offer the greatest protection from both UVA and UVB exposure that can lead to an increased risk of skin cancer.

Sunscreen products that pass the broad spectrum test are allowed to be labeled as "Broad Spectrum." These "Broad Spectrum" sunscreens protect against both UVA and UVB rays. For "Broad Spectrum" sunscreens, the "Sun Protection Factor" or SPF also indicates the overall amount of protection provided. Broad Spectrum sunscreens with SPF values of 15 or higher help protect against not only sunburn, but also skin cancer and early skin aging when used as directed with other sun protection measures. These sun protection measures include limiting time in the sun and wearing protective clothing.

For sunscreen products labeled with SPF values but not as "Broad Spectrum," the SPF value indicates the amount of protection against sunburn only.

These testing and labeling requirements are necessary to provide consumers with the information they need to make informed choices when selecting sunscreens.

Q2. When will these changes take effect?
A. The Final Rule will take effect by the summer of 2012, but consumers may begin to see changes to sunscreen labels before the effective date.

Q3. What do consumers need to know when buying and using sunscreens?
A. Spending time in the sun increases a person's risk of skin cancer and early skin aging. To reduce these risks, consumers should regularly use a Broad Spectrum sunscreen with an SPF value of 15 or higher in combination with other protective measures such as:

- Limiting time in the sun, especially between the hours of 10 AM and 2 PM when the sun's rays are the strongest.
- Wearing clothing to cover skin exposed to the sun (long-sleeved shirts, pants, sunglasses, and broad-brimmed hats).
- Using a water resistant sunscreen if swimming or sweating.
- Reapplying sunscreen, even if it is labeled as water resistant, at least every 2 hours. (Water resistant sunscreens should be reapplied more often after swimming or sweating, according to the directions on the label.)

Q4. What are the main points of the new Final Rule?
A. The new final rule includes the following requirements:

- Broad Spectrum designation. Sunscreens that pass FDA's broad spectrum test procedure, which measures a product's UVA protection relative to its UVB protection, may be labeled as "Broad Spectrum SPF [*value*]" on the front label. For Broad Spectrum sunscreens, SPF values also indicate the amount or magnitude of overall protection. Broad Spectrum SPF products with SPF values higher than 15 provide greater protection and may claim additional uses, as described in the next bullet.

- Use claims. Only Broad Spectrum sunscreens with an SPF value of 15 or higher can claim to reduce the risk of skin cancer and early skin aging if used as directed with other sun protection measures. Non-Broad Spectrum sunscreens and Broad Spectrum sunscreens with an SPF value between 2 and 14 can only claim to help prevent sunburn.

- "Waterproof, "sweatproof" or "sunblock" claims. Manufacturers cannot label sunscreens as "waterproof" or "sweatproof," or identify their products as "sunblocks," because these claims overstate their effectiveness. Sunscreens also cannot claim to provide sun protection for more than 2 hours without reapplication or to provide protection immediately after application (for example-- "instant protection") without submitting data to support these claims and obtaining FDA approval.

- Water resistance claims. Water resistance claims on the front label must indicate whether the sunscreen remains effective for 40 minutes or 80 minutes while swimming or sweating, based on standard testing. Sunscreens that are not water resistant must include a direction instructing consumers to use a water resistant sunscreen if swimming or sweating.

- Drug Facts. All sunscreens must include standard "Drug Facts" information on the back and/or side of the container.

Q5. What does the Proposed Rule address?

A. The proposed rule, if finalized, would limit the maximum SPF value on sunscreen labels to "50 +" because there is not sufficient data to show that products with SPF values higher than 50 provide greater protection for users than products with SPF values of 50.

The proposed regulation (PDF - 197KB)1 is available for public comment until September 15, 2011.

Q6. What is the purpose of the Advance Notice of Proposed Rulemaking (ANPR)?

A. The Advance Notice of Proposed Rulemaking (ANPR) allows the public a period of time to comment on regulations FDA may pursue as part of future rulemaking. In developing regulations for over-the-counter (OTC) sunscreens, FDA has not previously specified to which dosage forms the regulations would apply. Therefore, FDA is requesting additional data relating to sunscreen products in specific dosage forms to further our understanding of how dosage forms affect safety and effectiveness.

For example, the ANPR invites public comment on possible directions for use of and warnings for sunscreen sprays, as well as supporting data or information for sprays and other sunscreen dosage forms including lotions, oils, sticks, gels, butters, ointments, creams, and pastes. The ANPR also explains how interested parties can supply information for FDA to consider other dosage forms, including powders, towelettes, body washes, and shampoos.

Q7. Why is the Advance Notice of Proposed Rulemaking (ANPR) requesting additional data on sunscreen products in the form of sprays?

A. Currently, the record (data and information) about sunscreens in spray dosage forms is not comparable to that for sunscreens in other dosage forms such as oils, creams, and lotions. The manner of application differs significantly between sprays and these other dosage forms. Therefore, we are requesting additional data to address questions of effectiveness and safety that arise from differences in the manner of application.

Q8. What is included in the Draft Guidance for Industry?

A. The Draft Guidance for Industry is an enforcement guidance that includes information to help sunscreen product manufacturers understand how to label and test their products in light of the new Final Rule, the Proposed Rule, and the Advance Notice of Proposed Rulemaking (ANPR).

Q9. Why isn't FDA finalizing all the proposed sunscreen changes under one rule?

A. FDA is finalizing those changes that are based on proposals it made in earlier stages of rulemaking, including a 2007 proposed rule, on which it already received public comment. Those comments also helped to inform the Agency's thinking about additional aspects of sunscreen regulation, which in turn gave rise to the Proposed Rule and Advance Notice of Proposed Rulemaking (ANPR). The regulatory process requires FDA to give public notice and opportunity for comment before finalizing additional changes, which also gives the public and Agency an opportunity to further develop the record (data and information) on safety and effectiveness.

Q10. Where can I find more information on these various regulatory actions?

A. On June 14, 2011, FDA published the new sunscreen Final Rule (PDF - 485KB)2, the Proposed Rule (PDF - 197KB)3, the Advance Notice of Proposed Rulemaking (ANPR) (PDF - 187KB)4 and the notice of availability of the Draft Guidance for Industry (PDF - 217KB)5 in the *Federal Register*. The draft guidance, *Enforcement Policy – OTC Sunscreen Drug Products Marketed Without an Approved Application* (PDF - 132KB)6, is also available.

Source: FDA Website. Questions and Answers: FDA announces new requirements for over-the-counter (OTC) sunscreen products marketed in the U.S. Available at: http://www.fda.gov/Drugs/ ResourcesForYou/Consumers/BuyingUsingMedicineSafely/ UnderstandingOver-the-CounterMedicines/ucm258468.htm. Accessed June 15, 2011.

271

References

1. CDC Website. Seven Safety Suggestions for Summer Work: #5 Slather yourself in sunscreen. Available at: www.cdc.gov/Features/WorkingOutdoors/. Accessed December 21, 2010.
2. Chemical & Engineering News Website. Science & Technology. Sunscreens: Active ingredients prevent skin damage. June 24, 2002. 80(25):38. Available at: www.pubs.acs.org/cen/whatstuff/stuff/8025sunscreens.html. Accessed May 12, 2011.
   Happi Household and Personal Products Industry Website. Sunscreen sales have room to grow. Available at: www.happi.com/news/2010/02/15/sunscreen_sales_have_room_to_grow. Accessed May 12, 2011.
3. Random History Website. Protecting your skin: The history of sunscreen. Available at: www.randomhistory.com/2009/04/28_sunscreen.html.
   Shaath N. *Sunscreens: Regulations and Commercial Development*. 3rd ed. Informa Healthcare. 2005. Page 4.
4. Himaya Website. A Brief History of Sunscreens. Available at: www.himaya.com/faq/sunscreen_history.html. Accessed 5/27/11.
   About.com Website. Moore D. Allergies to Sunscreens. Available at: http://allergies.about.com/od/contactdermatitis/a/sunscreens.htm. Accessed June 17, 2011.
   Medscape Website. Scheuer E, Warshaw E. Sunscreen Allergy: A Review of Epidemiology, Clinical Characteristics, and Responsible Allergens. Available at: www.medscape.com/viewarticle/528577_7. Accessed June 17, 2011.
5. Heart Spring Website. Beck S. The history of sunscreen skin care. Available at: www.heartspring.net/skin_care_skin_cancer_sunscreen.html. Accessed December 20, 2010.
6. Himaya Website. A Brief History of Sunscreens. Available at: www.himaya.com/faq/sunscreen_history.html. Accessed 5/27/11.
   About.com Website. Moore D. Allergies to Sunscreens. Available at: http://allergies.about.com/od/contactdermatitis/a/sunscreens.htm. Accessed June 17, 2011.
   Medscape Website. Scheuer E, Warshaw E. Sunscreen Allergy: A Review of Epidemiology, Clinical Characteristics, and Responsible Allergens. Available at: www.medscape.com/viewarticle/528577_7. Accessed June 17, 2011.
7. Hodges ND, Moss SH, Davies DJ. Evidence for increased genetic damage due to the presence of a sunscreen agent, para-aminobenzoic acid, during irradiation with near ultraviolet light [proceedings]. *J Pharm Pharmacol*. 1976. 28 Suppl:53P.
8. Knowland J, McKenzie EA, McHugh PJ, Cridland NA. Sunlight-induced mutagenicity of a common sunscreen ingredient. FEBS Lett. 1993. 324(3):309-313.
9. Flindt-Hansen H, Thune P, Eeg-Larsen T. The effect of short-term application of PABA on photocarcinogenesis. Acta Derm Venereol. 1990. 70(1):72-75.

10. Kumakiri M, Hashimoto K, Willis I. Biologic changes due to long-wave ultraviolet irradiation on human skin: ultrastructural study. *J Invest Dermatol*. 1977. 69(4):392-400.
11. ChemEurope.com Website. Avobenzone. Available at: www.chemeurope.com/ en/encyclopedia/Avobenzone.html. Accessed June 17, 2011.
12. Cancer Org Website. Skin Cancer: Basal and Squamous Cell Overview. www. cancer.org/Cancer/SkinCancer-BasalandSquamousCell/OverviewGuide/ skin-cancer-basal-and-squamous-cell-overview-what-is-skin-cancer. Accessed June 17, 2011.
Histology at Southern Illinois University School of Medicine Website. Introduction to Skin Histology. Available at: www.siumed.edu/~dking2/ intro/skin.htm#epidermis. Accessed April 27, 2011.
13. eMedicine Website. Amirlak B. Skin anatomy. Available at: http://emedicine. medscape.com/article/1294744-overview. Accessed 5/27/10.
14. Hill HZ. The function of melanin or six blind people examine an elephant. *Bioessays*. 1992. 14(1):49-56. Available at: www.drproctor.com/os/ melaninfunction.htm.
15. Bastuji-Garin S. Diepgen TL. Cutaneous malignant melanoma, sun exposure, and sunscreen use: epidemiological evidence. *Br J Dermatol*. 2002. 146(Suppl. 61):24–30. Review.
16. World Health Organization Website: The World Health Organization recommends that no person under 18 should use a sunbed. Available at: www.who.int/ mediacentre/news/notes/2005/np07/en/index.html. Accessed November 8, 2010.
17. Jemal A, Devesa SS, Hartge P, Tucker MA. Recent trends in cutaneous melanoma incidence among whites in the United States. J Natl Cancer Inst. 2001. 93(9):678-683. Available at: http://jnci.oxfordjournals.org/ content/93/9/678.full
Ries LA, Wingo PA, Miller DS, et al. The annual report to the nation on the status of cancer, 1973-1997, with a special section on colorectal cancer. *Cancer*. 2000. 88(10):2398-2424.
18. Jemal A, Devesa SS, Hartge P, Tucker MA. Recent trends in cutaneous melanoma incidence among whites in the United States. *J Natl Cancer Inst*. 2001. 93(9):678-683. Available at: http://jnci.oxfordjournals.org/ content/93/9/678.full
National Cancer Insititute Website. Cancer Statistics: Fast Facts. Available at: www.seer.cancer.gov/faststats/selections.php?#Output. Accessed February 25, 2011.
19. Maine Cancer Registry Website. Melanoma: Risk Factors, Prevention & Early Detection. Available at: www.maine.gov/dhhs/bohdcfh/mcr/prevent/ melanoma.htm. Accessed February 5, 2011.
Jemal A, Devesa SS, Hartge P, Tucker MA. Recent trends in cutaneous melanoma incidence among whites in the United States. J Natl Cancer Inst. 2001. 93(9):678-683. Available at: http://jnci.oxfordjournals.org/ content/93/9/678.full.
Ries LA, Wingo PA, Miller DS, et al. The annual report to the nation on the status of cancer, 1973-1997, with a special section on colorectal cancer. *Cancer*. 2000. 88(10):2398-2424.
20. CDC Website. National Program of Cancer Registries (NPCR): United States Cancer Statistics (USCS). Available at: http://apps.nccd.cdc.gov/uscs/ toptencancers.aspx. Accessed June 17, 2011.

Jemal A, Murray T, Samuels A, Ghafoor A, Ward E, Thun MJ. Cancer statistics, 2003. *CA Cancer J Clin*. 2003. 53(1):5-26.

21. Rigel DS. The effect of sunscreen on melanoma risk. *Dermatol Clin*. 2002. 20:601-606.

National Cancer Institute (USA) Website. SEER stat fact sheets: Melanoma of the skin. Available at: www.seer.cancer.gov/statfacts/html/melan.html. Accessed December 20, 2010.

22. National Cancer Institute Website. Cancer Statistics: Fast Facts. Available at: http://seer.cancer.gov/faststats/selections.php?series=cancer. Accessed June 2, 2011.

National Cancer Institute (USA) Website. SEER stat fact sheets: Melanoma of the skin. Available at: www.seer.cancer.gov/statfacts/html/melan.html. (All cancers - Table 2.5 and Melanoma of the skin – Table 16.5) Accessed December 20, 2010

Medscape Website. Epidemiological Trends of Cutaneous Malignant Melanoma: Incidence of Cutaneous Malignant Melanoma. Available at: www.medscape.com/viewarticle/470300_2. Accessed February 5, 2011.

Altekruse SF, Kosary CL, Krapcho M, et al. SEER Cancer Statistics Review, 1975-2007, National Cancer Institute. Available at: www.seer.cancer.gov/csr/1975_2007/, based on November 2009 SEER data submission, posted to the SEER Website, 2010. Accessed May 3, 2011.

23. Strouse JJ, Fears TR, Tucker MA, Wayne AS. Pediatric melanoma: risk factor and survival analysis of the surveillance, epidemiology and end results database. *J Clin Oncol*. 2005. 23:4735-4741.

24. Linos E, Swetter SM, Cockburn MG, Colditz GA, Clarke CA. Increasing burden of melanoma in the United States. *J Invest Dermatol*. 2009. 129(7):1666–1674.

25. Lee KC, Weinstock MA. Melanoma is up: are we up to this challenge? *J Invest Dermatol*. 129(7): 1604-1606.

26. Buljan M, Rajacić N, Vurnek Zivković M, Blajić I, Kusić Z, Situm M. Epidemiological data on melanoma from the referral centre in Croatia (2002-2007). *Coll Antropol*. 2008. 32(Suppl 2):47-51.

27. Garbe C, Leiter U. Melanoma epidemiology and trends. 2009. *Clin Dermatol*. 27(1):3–9.

28. World Health Organization Website: The World Health Organization recommends that no person under 18 should use a sunbed. Available at: www.who.int/mediacentre/news/notes/2005/np07/en/index.html. Accessed June 1, 2011.

29. Garbe C, Leiter U. Melanoma epidemiology and trends. 2009. *Clin Dermatol*. 27(1):3–9.

30. Antoniou C, Kosmadak MG, Stratigos AJ, Katsambas AD. Sunscreens – what's important to know. J Eur Acad Derm Venereology. 2008. 22(9):1110–1119. Epub 2008 Aug 18. DOI: 10.1111/j.1468-3083.2007.02580.

31. Garland CF, Garland FC, Gorham ED. Rising trends in melanoma. An hypothesis concerning sunscreen effectiveness. *Ann Epidemiol*. 1993. 3(1):103-110.

32. Gloster HM Jr, Brodland DG. The epidemiology of skin cancer. *Dermatol Surg*. 1996. 22(3):217–226.

33. National Cancer Institute (USA) Website. SEER training modules: Layers of the skin. Available at: www.training.seer.cancer.gov/melanoma/anatomy/layers.html. Accessed June 1, 2011.

34. Parker SL, Tong T, Bolden S, Wingo PA. Cancer statistics, 1996. *CA Cancer J Clin*. 1996. 46(1):5-27.

Miller DL, Weinstock MA. Nonmelanoma skin cancer in the United States: incidence. *J Am Acad Dermatol*. 1994. 30:774-778.

Rigel D, Friedman RJ, and Kopf AW. Lifetime risk for development of skin cancer in U.S. population: Current estimate is now 1 in 5. *J Am Acad Dermatol*. 1996. 35(6):1012-1013.

National Cancer Institute Website. Fraser MC, Hartge P. Melanoma of the Skin. Available at: http://rex.nci.nih.gov/NCI_Pub_Interface/raterisk/risks163. html. Accessed June 13, 2011.

35. Christenson LJ, Borrowman TA, Vachon CM, et al. Incidence of basal cell and squamous cell carcinomas in a population younger than 40 years. *JAMA*. 2005. 294(6):681-690.

36. Gloster HM Jr, Brodland DG. The epidemiology of skin cancer. *Dermatol Surg*. 1996. 22(3):217–226.

Gray DT, Suman VJ, Su WP, Clay RP, Harmsen WS, Roenigk RK. Trends in the population-based incidence of squamous cell carcinoma of the skin first diagnosed between 1984 and 1992. *Arch Dermatol*. 1997. 133(6):735–740.

37. Bulliard JL, Panizzon RG, Levi F. Epidemiology of epithelial skin cancers [abstract]. *Rev Med Suisse*. 2009. 5(200):882, 884-888.

38. Situm M, Vurnek Zivkovie M, Dediol I, Zeljko Penavie J, Simie D. Knowledge and attitudes towards sun protection in Croatia. *Coll Antropol*. 2010. 34(Suppl. 1):141–146.

39. Buljan M, Rajacić N, Vurnek Zivković M, Blajić I, Kusić Z, Situm M. Epidemiological data on melanoma from the referral centre in Croatia (2002-2007). *Coll Antropol*. 2008. 32(Suppl 2):47-51.

40. Tarbuk A, Grancarić AM, Situm M, Martinis M. UV clothing and skin cancer. *Coll Antropol*. 2010. 34(Suppl 2):179-183.

41. Handel AE, Ramagopalan SV. Correspondence letter (April 17). The questionable effectiveness of sunscreen. *Lancet*. 2010. 376(9736):161-162. Author reply on 162. Comment on 375(9715):673-685.

42. Random History Website. Protecting your skin: The history of sunscreen. Available at: www.randomhistory.com/2009/04/28_sunscreen.html.

43. Web Archive Website. Handbook on Industrial Laser Safety: Wavelength Considerations. Available at: http://web.archive.org/web/20071028072110/http://info.tuwien.ac.at/iflt/safety/section1/1_1_1.htm. Accessed June 4, 2011.

Lumalier Website. UV Spectrum. Available at: www.lumalier.com/why-uv-works/the-uv-spectrum.html. Accessed June 4, 2011.

44. wiseGEEK Website. What is ultraviolet light? Available at: www.wisegeek.com/what-is-ultraviolet-light.htm. Accessed December 20, 2010.

Escobedo João F, et al., Ratios of UV, PAR and NIR components to global solar radiation measured at Botucatu site in Brazil, Renewable Energy. 2010. doi:10.1016/j.renene.2010.06.018 (Article in Press).

World Health Organization Website. UV radiation. Available at: www.who.int/uv/faq/whatisuv/en/index2.html. Accessed June 4, 2011.

National Toxicology Program Website. Ultraviolet (UV) Radiation, Broad Spectrum and UVA, UVB, and UVC. Available at: http://ntp.niehs.nih.gov/index.cfm?objectid=BD4CD88D-F1F6-975E-792094AC1CE4B062. Accessed June 4, 2011.

Jackson Medical Park Website. Booras CH. SPF, UVB and UVA Protection Explained. Available at: www.axmed.com/articles/wellness/spf.htm. Accessed June 14, 2011.

45. Science Daily Website. Sunscreen in a Pill: Dermatologists Discover Sun Protection under the Sea. Available at: www.sciencedaily.com/videos/2007/1108-sunscreen_in_a_pill.htm. Accessed January 25, 2011.

46. Jackson Medical Park Website. Booras CH. SPF, UVB and UVA Protection Explained. Available at: www.axmed.com/articles/wellness/spf.htm. Accessed June 14, 2011.

   eMedicine Website. Levy SB, Elston DM. Sunscreens and Photoprotection: Active Sunscreen Ingredients Overview. Available at: http://emedicine.medscape.com/article/1119992-overview#aw2aab6b4. Accessed June 4, 2011.

47. FDA Website. Questions and Answers: FDA announces new requirements for over-the-counter (OTC) sunscreen products marketed in the U.S. Available at: www.fda.gov/Drugs/ResourcesForYou/Consumers/BuyingUsingMedicineSafely/UnderstandingOver-the-CounterMedicines/ucm258468.htm. Accessed June 15, 2011.

   EPA Website. Sunscreen: The Burning Facts. Available at: www.epa.gov/sunwise/doc/sunscreen.pdf. Accessed June 4, 2011.

48. CDC Website. Seven Safety Suggestions for Summer Work: #5 Slather yourself in sunscreen. Available at: www.cdc.gov/Features/WorkingOutdoors/. Accessed December 21, 2010.

49. Genetics Home Reference Website. Reative Oxygen Species. Available at: www.ghr.nlm.nih.gov/glossary=reactiveoxygenspecies. Accessed June 1, 2011.

50. Hanson KM, Gratton E, Bardeen CJ. Sunscreen enhancement of UV-induced reactive oxygen species in the skin. *Free Radic Biol Med*. 2006. 41(8):1205-1212. Epub 2006 Jul 6.

51. Science Daily Website. Sunscreen in a pill: dermatologists discover sun protection under the sea. Available at: www.sciencedaily.com/videos/2007/1108-sunscreen_in_a_pill.htm. Accessed January 25, 2011.

   Rietjens SJ, Bast A, de Vente J, Haenen GR. The olive oil antioxidant hydroxytyrosol efficiently protects against the oxidative stress-induced impairment of the NObullet response of isolated rat aorta. *Am J Physiol Heart Circ Physiol*. 2007. 292(4):H1931-1936. Epub 2006 Dec 15.

   Hanson KM, Gratton E, Bardeen CJ. Sunscreen enhancement of UV-induced reactive oxygen species in the skin. *Free Radic Biol Med*. 2006. 41(8):1205-1212. Epub 2006 Jul 6.

   Medicine Net Website. Definition of reactive oxygen species. Available at: www.medterms.com/script/main/art.asp?articlekey=26097. Accessed December 21, 2010.

   Shapira N. Nutritional approach to sun protection: a suggested complement to external strategies. *Nutr Rev*. 68(2):75–86.

   Sander CS, Hamm F, Elsner P, Thiele JJ. Oxidative stress in malignant melanoma and non-melanoma skin cancer. *Br J Dermatol*. 2003. 148(5):913–922.

   Bossi O, Gartsbein M, Leitges M, Kuroki T, Grossman S, Tennenbaum T. UV irradiation increases ROS production via PKCdelta signaling in primary murine fibroblasts. *J Cell Biochem*. 2008. 105(5):194–207.

   Setlow RB, Grist E, Thompson K, Woodhead AD. Wave-lengths effective in induction of malignant melanoma. *Proc Natl Acad Sci USA*. 1993. 90(14):6666–6670.

Applegate LA, Luscher P, Tyrrell RM. Induction of heme oxygenase: a general response to oxidant stress in cultured mammalian cells. *Cancer Res.* 1991. 51(3):974–978. Cited in Shapira N. Nutritional approach to sun protection: a suggested complement to external strategies. *Nutr Rev.* 68(2):75–86.

Picardo M, Grammatico P, Roccella F, et al. Imbalance in the antioxidant pool in melanoma cells and normal melanocytes from patients with melanoma. *J Invest Dermatol.* 1996. 107(3):322–326.

52. Moyal DD, Fourtanier AM. Broad-spectrum sunscreens provide better protection from solar ultraviolet-simulated radiation and natural sunlight-induced immunosuppression in human beings. *J Am Acad Dermatol.* 2008. 58(5 Suppl 2):S149-154.

53. Young AR. Are broad-spectrum sunscreens necessary for immunoprotection? Review. *J Invest Dermatol.* 2003. 121(4):ix–x.

Society of Cosmetic Scientists Website. Hewitt JP. Suncare Formulating Strategies in the Changing Regulatory Environment. Available at: www.scss.org.sg/docs/JPHewittSCSS2008%20UVA.pdf. Accessed June 17, 2011.

FDA Website. Questions and Answers: FDA announces new requirements for over-the-counter (OTC) sunscreen products marketed in the U.S. Available at: www.fda.gov/Drugs/ResourcesForYou/Consumers/BuyingUsingMedicineSafely/UnderstandingOver-the-CounterMedicines/ucm258468.htm. Accessed June 15, 2011.

54. Agar NS, Halliday GM, Barnetson RS, Ananthaswamy HN, Wheeler M, Jones AM. The basal layer in human squamous tumors harbors more UVA than UVB fingerprint mutations: a role for UVA in human skin carcinogenesis. Proc Natl Acad Sci U S A. 2004. 101(14):4954-4959. Epub 2004 Mar 23.

Setlow RB, Grist E, Thompson K, Woodhead AD. Wave-lengths effective in induction of malignant melanoma. *Proc Natl Acad Sci USA.* 1993. 90(14):6666–6670.

55. Callaghan TM, Wilhelm KP. A review of ageing and an examination of clinical methods in the assessment of ageing skin. Part I: Cellular and molecular perspectives of skin ageing. *Int J Cosmet Sci.* 2008. 30(5):313-322.

Article Base Website. Understanding How Collagen Functions and How It Benefits You. Available at: www.articlesbase.com/health-articles/understanding-how-collagen-functions-and-how-it-benefits-you-310875.html. Accessed April 27, 2011.

Histology at Southern Illinois University School of Medicine Website. Introduction to Skin Histology. Available at: www.siumed.edu/~dking2/intro/skin.htm#epidermis. Accessed April 27, 2011.

Young AR. Are broad-spectrum sunscreens necessary for immunoprotection? Review. *J Invest Dermatol.* 2003. 121(4):ix–x.

Antoniou C, Kosmadak MG, Stratigos AJ, Katsambas AD. Sunscreens – what's important to know. J Eur Acad Derm Venereology. 2008. 22(9):1110–1119. Epub 2008 Aug 18. DOI: 10.1111/j.1468-3083.2007.02580.x

Kohen R. Skin antioxidants: their role in aging and in oxidative stress – new approaches for their evaluation. Biomed Pharmacother. 1999. 53(4):181–192. Cited in Shapira N. Nutritional approach to sun protection: a suggested complement to external strategies. *Nutr Rev.* 68(2):75–86.

56. Science Daily Website. Sunscreens Can Danage Skin, Reserchers Find. Available at: www.sciencedaily.com/releases/2006/08/060828211528.htm. Accessed June 26, 2011.

Autier P. Sunscreen abuse for intentional sun exposure. *Br J Dermatol.* 2009. 161(Suppl 3):40-45.

Marrot L, Meunier JR. Skin DNA photodamage and its biological consequences. J Am Acad Dermatol. 2008. 58(5 Suppl 2):S139–S148.

57. Scribd Website. Using TiO$_2$ and ZnO for balance UV protection. Available at: http://www.scribd.com/doc/50005737/Using-TiO$_2$-and-ZnO-for-balanced-UV-protection. Accessed June 26, 2011.

58. Scribd Website. Using TiO$_2$ and ZnO for balance UV protection. Available at: http://www.scribd.com/doc/50005737/Using-TiO$_2$-and-ZnO-for-balanced-UV-protection. Accessed June 26, 2011.

FDA Website. Shao Y, Delrieu P. Perspectives on Supplying Attneuation Grades of Titanium Dioxide and Zinc Oxide for Sunscreen Applications. Available at: www.fda. gov/ScienceResearch/SpecialTopics/Nanotechnology/NanotechnologyTaskForce/ ucm119516.htm. Accessed June 26, 2011.

Newman MD, Stotland M, Ellis JI. The safety of nanosized particles in titanium dioxide and zinc oxide based sunscreens. *J Am Acad Dermatol.* 2009. 61(4):685-692. Epub 2009 Jul 31.

wiseGEEK Website. What is the history of sunscreens? Available at: www. wisegeek.com/what-is-the-history-of-sunscreen.htm. Accessed December 20, 2010.

59. Smart Skin Care Website. Chemical UVA+UVB sunscreen/sunblock - Bisoctrizole (Tinosorb M). Available at: www.smartskincare.com/ skinprotection/sunblocks/sunblock_bisoctrizole.html. Accessed December 21, 2010.

60. Ashby J, Tinwell H, Plautz J, Twomey K, Lefevre PA. Lack of binding to isolated estrogen or androgen receptors, and inactivity in the immature rat uterotrophic assay, of the ultraviolet sunscreen filters Tinosorb M-active and Tinosorb S. *Regul Toxicol Pharmacol.* 2001. 34(3):287-291.

61. Wikipedia Website. Avobenzone. Available at: http://en.wikipedia.org/wiki/ Avobenzone. Accessed December 21, 2010.

62. FDA Website. Phototoxicology. Available at: www.fda.gov/AboutFDA/ CentersOffices/nctr/WhatWeDo/NCTRCentersofExcellence/ucm078968. htm. Accessed February 7, 2011.

63. FDA: Food and Drug Administration (U.S.) Website. Department of Health Memorandum: Summary of Pediatric Safety Data used for Approval of Anthelios 40 NDA 22-009. Available at: www.fda.gov/ downloads/AdvisoryCommittees/CommitteesMeetingMaterials/ PediatricAdvisoryCommittee/UCM204843.pdf. Accessed December 21, 2010.

FDA: Food and Drug Administration (U.S.) Website. CFR–Code of Federal Regulations Title 21. Available at: www.accessdata.fda.gov/scripts/cdrh/ cfdocs/cfcfr/CFRSearch.cfm?CFRPart=352&showFR=1. Accessed April 27, 2011.

64. Donnelly B. Fox News: Health Center Website. FDA Set to Slather Us With New Sunscreen Regulations, But Will They Stick? Available at: www.foxnews. com/health/2010/07/02/fda-set-slather-new-sunscreen-regulations-stick/. Accessed December 21, 2010.

65. FDA: Food and Drug Administration (U.S.) Website. Phototoxicology. Available at: www.fda.gov/AboutFDA/CentersOffices/nctr/WhatWeDo/ NCTRCentersofExcellence/ucm078968.htm. Accessed February 7, 2011.

66. FDA Website. Department of Health Memorandum: Summary of Pediatric Safety Data used for Approval of Anthelios 40 NDA 22-009. Available at: www.fda.gov/downloads/AdvisoryCommittees/CommitteesMeetingMaterials/PediatricAdvisoryCommittee/UCM204843.pdf. Accessed December 21, 2010.

67. Donnelly B. Fox News: Health Center Website. FDA Set to Slather Us With New Sunscreen Regulations, But Will They Stick? Available at: www.foxnews.com/health/2010/07/02/fda-set-to-slather-new-sunscreen-regulations-stick/. Accessed December 21, 2010.

68. FDA Website. Questions and Answers: FDA announces new requirements for over-the-counter (OTC) sunscreen products marketed in the U.S. Available at: www.fda.gov/Drugs/ResourcesForYou/Consumers/BuyingUsingMedicineSafely/UnderstandingOver-the-CounterMedicines/ucm258468.htm. Accessed June 15, 2011.

69. GPO Website. Food and Drug Administration, HHS § 352.72: Composition of Preparation A and Preparation B of the Standard Sunscreen. Available at: http://edocket.access.gpo.gov/cfr_2006/aprqtr/pdf/21cfr352.72.pdf. Accessed December 21, 2010.

Chapin R, Gulati D, Mounce R. 2-Hydroxy-4-methoxybenzophenone. Environ Health Perspect. 1997. 105(Supplement 1):313-314. Available at: www.ncbi.nlm.nih.gov/pmc/articles/PMC1470294/pdf/envhper00326-0308.pdf.

Jarry H, Christoffel J, Rimoldi G, Koch L, Wuttke W. Multi-organic endocrine disrupting activity of the UV screen benzophenone 2 (BP2) in ovariectomized adult rats after 5 days treatment. *Toxicology*. 2004. 205(1-2):87–93.

Schlecht C, Klammer H, Frauendorf H. Wuttke W, Jarry H. Pharmacokinetics and metabolism of benzophenone 2 in the rat. *Toxicology*. 2008. 245(1-2):11-17. Epub 2007 Dec 27.

Schlumpf M, Cotton B, Conscience M, Haller V, Steinmann B, Lichtensteiger W. In vitro and in vivo estrogenicity of UV screens. *Environ Health Perspect*. 2001. 109(3):239–244.

Schlumpf M, Schmid P, Durrer S, et. al. Endocrine activity and developmental toxicity of cosmetic UV filters–an update. *Toxicology*. 2004. 205:113–122.

Schlumpf M, Durrer S, Faass O, et al. Developmental toxicity of UV filters and environmental exposure: a review. *Int J Androl*. 2008. 31(2):144-151. Epub 2008 Jan 10.

Durrer S, Ehnes C, Fuetsch M, Maerkel K, Schlumpf M, Lichtensteiger W. Estrogen sensitivity of target genes and expression of nuclear receptor co-regulators in rat prostate after pre- and postnatal exposure to the ultraviolet filter 4-methylbenzylidene camphor. *Environ Health Perspect*. 2007. 115(Suppl 1):42–50.

Hofkamp L, Bradley S, Tresguerres J, Lichtensteiger W, Schlumpf M, Timms B. Region-specific growth effects in the developing rat prostate following fetal exposure to estrogenic ultraviolet filters. *Environ Health Perspect*. 2008. 116(7):867–872.

Axelstad M, Boberg J, Hougaard KS, et al. Effects of pre-and postnatal exposure to the UV-filter Octyl Methoxycinnamate (OMC) on the reproductive, auditory and neurological development of rat offspring. *Toxicol Appl Pharmacol*. 2011. 250(3):278-290. Epub 2010 Nov 6.

70. CDC Website. Seven Safety Suggestions for Summer Work: #5 Slather yourself in sunscreen. Available at: www.cdc.gov/Features/WorkingOutdoors/. Accessed December 21, 2010.

Smart Skin Care Website. Chemical UVA+UVB sunscreen/sunblock - Bisoctrizole (Tinosorb M). Available at: www.smartskincare.com/ skinprotection/sunblocks/sunblock_bisoctrizole.html. Accessed December 21, 2010.

Antoniou C, Kosmadak MG, Stratigos AJ, Katsambas AD. Sunscreens – what's important to know. *J Eur Acad Derm Venereology.* 2008. 22(9):1110–1119. Epub 2008 Aug 18. DOI: 10.1111/j.1468-3083.2007.02580.x

Wikipedia Website. Sunscreen. Available at: http://en.wikipedia.org/wiki/ Sunscreen. Accessed December 21, 2010.

Interlude Medical Spa Website. Skin care products and mineral makeup Vancouver Washington. Available at: www.interludemedicalspa.net/home/ skin%20care%20products.html. Accessed February 7, 2011.

71. Young AR. Are broad-spectrum sunscreens necessary for immunoprotection? Review. *J Invest Dermatol.* 2003. 121(4):ix–x.

72. Society of Cosmetic Scientists Website. Hewitt JP. Suncare Formulating Strategies in the Changing Regulatory Environment. Available at: www. scss.org.sg/docs/JPHewittSCSS2008%20UVA.pdf. Accessed June 17, 2011.

FDA Website. Questions and Answers: FDA announces new requirements for over-the-counter (OTC) sunscreen products marketed in the U.S. Available at: www. fda.gov/Drugs/ResourcesForYou/Consumers/BuyingUsingMedicineSafely/ UnderstandingOver-the-CounterMedicines/ucm258468.htm. Accessed June 15, 2011.

73. Nichols JA, Katiyar SK. Skin photoprotection by natural polyphenols: anti-inflammatory, antioxidant and DNA repair mechanisms. *Arch Dermatol Res.* 2010. 302(2):71-83. Epub 2009 Nov 7.

74. Spijker GT, Schuttelaar MLA, Barkema L, Velders A, Coenraads PJ. Anaphylaxis caused by topical application of a sunscreen containing benzophenone-3. *Contact Dermatitis.* 2008. 59(4):248–249.

Landers M, Law S, Storrs FJ. Contact urticaria, allergic contact dermatitis, and photoallergic contact dermatitis from oxybenzone. *Am J Contact Dermat.* 2003. 14(1):33–34.

Yesudian P D, King CM. Severe contact urticaria and anaphylaxis from benzophenone-3 (2-hydroxy 4-methoxy benzophenone). *Contact Dermatitis.* 2002. 46(1):55–56.

Emonet S, Pasche-Koo F, Perin-Minisini M J, Hauser C. Anaphylaxis to oxybenzone, a frequent constituent of sunscreens. *J Allergy Clin Immunol.* 2001. 107(3):556–557.

75. Armeni T, Damiani E, Battino M, Greci L, Principato G. Lack of in vitro protection by a common sunscreen ingredient on UVA-induced cytotoxicity in keratinocytes. *Toxicology.* 2004. 203(1-3):165-178.

76. Paris C, Lhiaubet-Vallet V, Jimenez O, Trullas C, Miranda MA. A blocked diketo form of avobenzone: photostability, photosensitizing properties and triplet quenching by a triazine-derived UVB-filter. *Photochem Photobiol.* 85(1):178–184. Epub 2008 Jul 30.

77. Kobo Products Inc. Website. Nguyen U, Scholossman D. Stability Study of Avobenzone with Inorganic Sunscreens. Available at: www.koboproductsinc. com/Downloads/NYSCC-Avobenzone.pdf. Accessed March 20, 2011.

78. Tomecki MH. OTC product: Anthelios SX. *J Am Pharm Assoc* (2003). 2007. 47(5):672.

79. Giacomoni PU, Teta L, Najdek L. Sunscreens: the impervious path from theory to practice. *Photochem Photobiol Sci.* 2010. 9(4):524–529.

80. CIR (Cosmetic Ingredient Review). Final report on the safety assessment of benzophenones-1, 3, 4, 5, 9, and 11. *J Am Col Toxicol.* 1983. 2(5):42.

81. Zero Breast Cancer Website. Barlow J, Johnson JA. Breast Cancer and the Environment Research Centers: Early Life Exposure to Phenols and Breast Cancer Risk in Later Years. Fact Sheet on Phenols. Available at: www. zerobreastcancer.org/research/bcerc_factsheets_phenols.pdf. Accessed December 28, 2010.

82. Kunz PY, Fent K. Multiple hormonal activities of UV filters and comparison of in vivo and in vitro estrogenic activity of ethyl-4-aminobenzoate in fish. *Aquat Toxicol.* 2006. 79(4):305-324. Epub 2006 Jun 30.

83. Chapin R, Gulati D, Mounce R. 2-Hydroxy-4-methoxybenzophenone. Environ Health Perspect. 1997. 105(Supplement 1):313-314. Available at: www. ncbi.nlm.nih.gov/pmc/articles/PMC1470294/pdf/envhper00326-0308.pdf.

84. Jarry H, Christoffel J, Rimoldi G, Koch L, Wuttke W. Multi-organic endocrine disrupting activity of the UV screen benzophenone 2 (BP2) in ovariectomized adult rats after 5 days treatment. *Toxicology.* 2004. 205(1-2):87–93.

85. Schlumpf M, Cotton B, Conscience M, Haller V, Steinmann B, Lichtensteiger W. In vitro and in vivo estrogenicity of UV screens. *Environ Health Perspect.* 2001. 109(3):239–244.

86. Schlumpf M, Schmid P, Durrer S, et. al. Endocrine activity and developmental toxicity of cosmetic UV filters–an update. *Toxicology.* 2004. 205:113–122.

87. Schlumpf M, Durrer S, Faass O, et al. Developmental toxicity of UV filters and environmental exposure: a review. *Int J Androl.* 2008. 31(2):144-151. Epub 2008 Jan 10.

88. Durrer S, Ehnes C, Fuetsch M, Maerkel K, Schlumpf M, Lichtensteiger W. Estrogen sensitivity of target genes and expression of nuclear receptor co-regulators in rat prostate after pre- and postnatal exposure to the ultraviolet filter 4-methylbenzylidene camphor. *Environ Health Perspect.* 2007. 115(Suppl 1):42–50.

89. Hofkamp L, Bradley S, Tresguerres J, Lichtensteiger W, Schlumpf M, Timms B. Region-specific growth effects in the developing rat prostate following fetal exposure to estrogenic ultraviolet filters. *Environ Health Perspect.* 2008. 116(7):867–872.

90. Axelstad M, Boberg J, Hougaard KS, et al. Effects of pre-and postnatal exposure to the UV-filter Octyl Methoxycinnamate (OMC) on the reproductive, auditory and neurological development of rat offspring. *Toxicol Appl Pharmacol.* 2010. doi:10.1016/j.taap.2010.10.031

91. Yoon Y, Ryu J, Oh J, Choi BG, Snyder SA. Occurrence of endocrine disrupting compounds, pharmaceuticals, and personal care products in the Han River (Seoul, South Korea). *Sci Total Environ.* 2010. 408(3):636-643. Epub 2009 Nov 8.

92. Poiger T. Buser HR, Balmaer M, Bergqvist PA, Muller MD. Occurrence of UV filter compounds from sunscreens in surface waters: regional mass balance in two Swiss lakes. *Chemosphere.* 55(7):951-963

93. Cuderman P, Health E. Determination of UV filters and antimicrobial agens in environmental water samples. *Anal Bioanal Chem.* 2007. 3887(4):1343-1350. Epub 2006 Nov 29.

94. Jeon HK, Chung Y, Ryu JC. *J Chromat A.* 2006. 113:192.

95. Langeford K, Thomas KV. Inputs of chemicals from recreational activities to the Norwegian coastal zone. In SETAC Europe 17th Annual Meeting. 2007. Porto Portugal.

96. Loraine GA, Pettigrove ME. *Environ Sci Technol*. 2006. 40:687.

97. Balmer ME, Buser HR, Müller MD, Poiger T. Occurrence of some organic UV filters in wastewater, in surface waters, and in fish from Swiss lakes. Environ. Sci. Technol. 2005, 39(4):953-962. Cited in Fent K, Kunz PY, Gomez E. UV filters in the aquatic environment induce hormonal effects and affect fertility and reproduction in fish. Endocrine disruptors: natural waters and fishes. *Chimia*. 2008. 62(5):368-375.

98. Nagtegaal M, Ternes TA, Baumann W. U UWSF-2. *Umweltchem Okotoxikol*. 1997. 9:79.

99. Buser HR, Balmer ME, Schmid P, Kohler M. Occurrence of UV filters 4-methylbenzylidene camphor and octocrylene in fish from various Swiss rivers with inputs from wastewater treatment plants. *Environ Sci Technol*. 2006. 40(5):1427-1431. Comment in: *Environ. Sci. Technol*. 2006, 40(5):1377-1378.

100. Plagellat C, Kupper T, Furrer R, de Alencastro LF, Grandjean D, Tarradellas J. Concentrations and specific loads of UV filters in sewage sludge originating from a monitoring network in Switzerland. *Chemosphere*. 2006 Feb;62(6):915-925. Epub 2005 Jul 5.

101. Balmer ME, Buser HR, Müller MD, Poiger T. Occurrence of some organic UV filters in wastewater, in surface waters, and in fish from Swiss lakes. *Environ Sci Technol*. 2005, 39(4):953-962. Cited in Fent K, Kunz PY, Gomez E. UV filters in the aquatic environment induce hormonal effects and affect fertility and reproduction in fish. Endocrine disruptors: natural waters and fishes. *Chimia*. 2008. 62(5):368-375.

102. Weisbrod CJ, Kunz PY, Zenker AK, Fent K. Effects of the UV filter benzophenone-2 on reproduction in fish. *Toxicol Appl Pharmacol*. 2007. 225(3):255-266. Epub 2007 Aug 17.

103. Coronado M, De Haro H, Deng X, Rempel MA, Lavado R, Schlenk D. Estrogenic activity and reproductive effects of the UV-filter oxybenzone (2-hydroxy-4-methoxyphenyl-methanone) in fish. *Aquat Toxicol*. 2008. 90(3):182–187. Epub 2008 Sep 10.

104. Kunz PY, Galicia HF, Fent K. Comparison of in vitro and in vivo estrogenic activity of UV filters in fish. *Toxicol Sci*. 2006. 90(2):349-361. Epub 2006 Jan 10.

105. Inui M, Adachi T, Takenaka S, et al. Effect of UV screens and preservatives on vitellogenin and choriogenin production in male medaka (Oryzias latipes). *Toxicology*. 2003. 194(1-2):43-50.

106. Kunz PY, Fent K. Multiple hormonal activities of UV filters and comparison of in vivo and in vitro estrogenic activity of ethyl-4-aminobenzoate in fish. *Aquat Toxicol*. 2006. 79(4):305-324. Epub 2006 Jun 30.

107. Molina-Molina JM, Escande A, Pillon A, Gomez E, et al. Profiling of benzophenone derivatives using fish and human estrogen receptor-specific in vitro bioassays. *Toxicol Appl Pharmacol*. 2008. 232(3):384-395. Epub 2008 Jul 29.

108. Kiparissis Y, Metcalfe TL, Balch GC, Metcalfe CD. Effects of the antiandrogens, vinclozolin and cyproterone acetate on gonadal development in the Japanese medaka (Oryzias latipes). *Aquat Toxicol*. 2003. 63(4):391-403. Abstract.

109. Okereke CS, Abdel-Rhaman MS, Friedman MA. Disposition of benzophenone-3 after dermal administration in male rats. *Toxicol Lett.* 1994. 73(2):113-122. Abstract.

110. Kunz PY, Fent K. Multiple hormonal activities of UV filters and comparison of in vivo and in vitro estrogenic activity of ethyl-4-aminobenzoate in fish. *Aquat Toxicol.* 2006. 79(4):305-324. Epub 2006 Jun 30.

111. Balmer ME, Buser HR, Müller MD, Poiger T. Occurrence of some organic UV filters in wastewater, in surface waters, and in fish from Swiss lakes. *Environ Sci Technol.* 2005, 39(4):953-962.

  Coronado M, De Haro H, Deng X, Rempel MA, Lavado R, Schlenk D. Estrogenic activity and reproductive effects of the UV-filter oxybenzone (2-hydroxy-4-methoxyphenyl-methanone) in fish. *Aquat Toxicol.* 2008. 90(3):182–187. Epub 2008 Sep 10.

112. Brian JV, Harris CA, Scholze M, et al. Evidence of estrogenic mixture effects on the reproductive performance of fish. *Environ Sci Technol.* 2007. 41(1):337-344.

113. Fent K, Kunz PY, Zenker A, Rapp M. A tentative environmental risk assessment of the UV-filters 3-(4-methylbenzylidene-camphor), 2-ethyl-hexyl-4-trimethoxycinnamate, benzophenone-3, benzophenone-4 and 3-benzylidene camphor. *Mar Environ Res.* 2010. 69(Suppl):S4–S6. Epub 2009 Nov 11.

114. Buser HR, Balmer ME, Schmid P, Kohler M. Occurrence of UV filters 4-methylbenzylidene camphor and octocrylene in fish from various Swiss rivers with inputs from wastewater treatment plants. Environ Sci Technol. 2006. 40(5):1427-1431. Comment in: *Environ Sci Technol.* 2006, 40(5):1377-1378.

115. Fent K, Zenker A, Rapp M. Widespread occurrence of estrogenic UV-filters in aquatic ecosystems in Switzerland. *Environ Pollut.* 2010. 158(5):1817-1824. Epub 2009 Dec 9. Abstract.

116. Chemical Book Website. Benzophenone (119-61-9). Available at: www.chemicalbook.com/ProductMSDSDetailCB5744679_EN.htm. Accessed February 7, 2011.

  JT Baker Website. MSDS: Benzophenone. Available at: www.jtbaker.com/msds/englishhtml/b1488.htm. Accessed December 29, 2010.

117. Benson HA. Assessment and clinical implications of absorption of sunscreens across skin. *Am J Clin Dermatol.* 2000. 1(4):217-224. Abstract.

118. Okereke CS, Kadry AM, Abdel-Rahman MS, Davis RA, Friedman MA. Metabolism of benzophenone-3 in rats. *Drug Metab Dispos.* 1993. 21(5):788-791.

119. Okereke CS, Abdel-Rhaman MS, Friedman MA. Disposition of benzophenone-3 after dermal administration in male rats. *Toxicol Lett.* 1994. 73(2):113-122. Abstract.

120. Kadry AM, Okereke CS, Abdel-Rahman MS, Friedman MA, Davis RA. Pharmacokinetics of benzophenone-3 after oral exposure in male rats. *J Appl Toxicol.* 1995. 15(2):97-102.

121. Gonzalez H, Farbrot A, Larkö O, Wennberg AM. Percutaneous absorption of the sunscreen benzophenone-3 after repeated whole-body applications, with and without ultraviolet irradiation. *Br J Dermatol.* 2006. 154(2):337-340.

122. Calafat AM, Wong LY, Ye X, Reidy JA, Needham LL. Concentrations of the sunscreen agent benzophenone-3 in residents of the United States: National Health and Nutrition Examination Survey 2003-2004. *Environ Health Perspect.* 2008. 116(7):893-897. Available at: www.medscape.com/viewarticle/577046.

123. Janjua NR, Kongshoj B, Andersson AM, Wulf HC. Sunscreens in human plasma and urine after repeated whole-body topical application. *J Eur Acad Dermatol Venereol.* 2008. 22(4):456-461. Epub 2008 Jan 23. Abstract.

124. Golmohammadzadeh S, Jaafarixx MR, Khalili N. Evaluation of liposomal and conventional formulations of octyl methoxycinnamate on human percutaneous absorption using the stripping method. *J Cosmet Sci.* 2008. 59(5):385-398.

Vettor M, Bourgeois S, Fessi H, et al. Skin absorption studies of octyl-methoxycinnamate loaded poly(D,L-lactide) nanoparticles: estimation of the UV filter distribution and release behaviour in skin layers. *J Microencapsul.* 2010. 27(3):253-262.

125. Durand L, Habran N, Henschel V, Amighi K. In vitro evaluation of the cutaneous penetration of sprayable sunscreen emulsions with high concentrations of UV filters. *Intl J Cosmet Sci.* 2009. 31(4):279–292.

126. Gupta VK, Zatz JL, Rerek M. Percutaneous absorption of sunscreens through micro-yucatan pig skin in vitro. Pharm Res. 1999. 16(10):1602-1607.

127. Wester RC, Noonan PK, Cole MP, Maibach HI. Percutaneous absorption of testosterone in the newborn rhesus monkey: comparison to the adult. *Pediatr Res.* 1977. 11(6):737–739.

West DP, Worobec S, Solomon LM. Pharmacology and toxicology of infant skin. *J Invest Dermatol.* 1981. 76(3):147–150.

128. Negreira N, Rodríguez I, Rubí E, Cela R. Determination of selected UV filters in indoor dust by matrix solid-phase dispersion and gas chromatography–tandem mass spectrometry. *J Chromatogr A.* 2009. 1216(31):5895-5902. Epub 2009 Jun 10.

129. Ye X, Kuklenyik Z, Needham LL, Calafat AM. Measuring environmental phenols and chlorinated organic chemicals in breast milk using automated on-line column-switching-high performance liquid chromatography-isotope dilution tandem mass spectrometry. *J Chromatogr B.* 2006. 831(1-2):110-115. Epub 2005 Dec 27.

130. Schlumpf M, Kypke K, Wittassek M, et. al. Exposure patterns of UV filters, fragrances, parabens, phthalates, organochlor pesticides, PBDEs, and PCBs in human milk: Correlation of UV filters with use of cosmetics. *Chemosphere.* 2010. 81(10):1171–1183. Epub 2010 Oct 27.

131. Chapin RE, Adams J, Boekelheide K, et al. NTP-CERHR expert panel report on the reproductive and developmental toxicity of bisphenol A. *Birth Defects Res B Dev Reprod Toxicol.* 2008. 83(3):157-395.

132. Bernal AJ, Jirtle RL Epigenomic disruption: the effects of early developmental exposures. *Birth Defects Res A Clin Mol Teratol.* 2010. 88(10):938-944.

133. Young AR. Are broad-spectrum sunscreens necessary for immunoprotection? Review. *J Invest Dermatol.* 2003. 121(4):ix–x.

134. Nishikawa M, Iwano H, Yanagisawa R, Koike N, Inoue H, Yokota H. Placental transfer of conjugated bisphenol A and subsequent reactivation in the rat fetus. *Environ Health Perspect.* 2010. 118(9):1196-1203. Epub 2010 Apr 9.

Balakrishnan B, Henare K, Thorstensen EB, Ponnampalam AP, Mitchell MD. Transfer of bisphenol A across the human placenta. *Am J Obstet Gynecol.* 2010. 202(4):393.e1-7.

135. Karnaky KJ. Diethylstilbestrol therapy; long period and high dosage Des therapy. *Med Times.* 1953. 81(5):315–317.

136. CDC Website. DES history. Available at: www.cdc.gov/des/consumers/about/history.html. Accessed December 29, 2010.

Giusti RM, Iwamoto K, Hatch EE. Diethylstilbestrol revisited: a review of the long-term health effects. *Ann Intern Med.* 1995. 122(10):778–788.

Dodds EC, Goldberg L, Larson W, Robinson R. Estrogenic activity of certain synthetic compounds. *Nature.* 1938. 141:247.

137. Metzler M. The metabolism of diethylstilbestrol. *CRC Crit Rev Biochem.* 1981. 10(3):171–212.

The DES Cancer Network Website: Timeline: A Brief History of DES (Diethylstilbestrol) www.descancer.org/timeline.html. Accessed May 3, 2011.

138. Raun AP, Preston RL. History of diethylstilbestrol use in cattle1 American Society of Animal Science. 2002. Available at: http://www.asas.org/Bios/Raunhist.pdf. Accessed May 3, 2011.

139. Herbst AL, Green TH Jr, Ulfelder H. Primary carcinoma of the vagina. An analysis of 68 cases. *Am J Obset Gynecol.* 1970. 106(2):210–218.

Herbst AL, Ulfelder H, Poskanzer DC. Adenocarcinoma of the vagina. Association of maternal stilbestrol therapy with tumor appearance in young women. *N Engl J Med.* 1971. 284(15):878–881.

Palmlund I. Exposure to a xenoestrogen before birth: the diethylstilbestrol experience. *J Psychosom Obstet Gynaecol.* 1996. 17(2):71–84.

Vessey MP, Fairweather DV, Norman-Smith B, Buckley J. A randomized double-blind controlled trial of the value of stilboestrol therapy in pregnancy: long-term follow-up of mothers and their offspring. *Br J Obstet Gynaecol.* 1983. 90(11):1007–1017.

Gill WB, Schumacher GF, Bibbo M. Structural and functional abnormalities in the sex organs of male offspring of mothers treated with diethylstilbestrol (DES). *J Reprod Med.* 1976. 16(4):147–153.

Palmer J R, Wise LA, Robboy SJ, et al. Hypospadias in sons of women exposed to diethylstilbestrol in utero. *Epidemiology.* 2005. 16(4):583–586.

Robboy SJ, Szyfelbein WM, Goellner JR, et al. Dysplasia and cytologic findings in 4,589 young women enrolled in diethylstilbestrol-adenosis (DESAD) project. *Am J Obset Gynecol.* 1981. 140(5):579–586.

Wilcox AJ, Baird DD, Weinberg CR, Hornsby PP, Herbst AL. Fertility in men exposed prenatally to diethylstilbestrol. *N Engl J Med.* 1995. 332(21):1411–1416.

Kalfa N, Paris F, Soyer-Gobillard MO, Daures JP, Sultan C. P Prevalence of hypospadias in grandsons of women exposed to diethylstilbestrol during pregnancy: a multigenerational national cohort study. *Fertil Steril.* 2011. [Epub ahead of print].

140. Patisaul HB, Adewale HB. Long-term effects of environmental endocrine disruptors on reproductive physiology and behavior. *Front Behav Neurosci.* 2009. 3(10):1-18.

Crews D, McLachlan JA. Epigenetics, evolution, endocrine disruption, health, and disease. Endocrinology. 2006. 147(6 Suppl):S4–S10. Epub 2006 May 11.

141. Wolf MS, Engel SM, Berkowitz GS, et al. Prenatal phenol and phthalate exposures and birth outcomes. *Environ Health Perspect.* 2008. 116(8):1092–1097.

142. Tetel MJ, Pfaff DW. Contributions of estrogen receptor-α and estrogen receptor-β to the regulation of behavior. *Biochim Biophys Acta.* 2010. 1800(10):1084–1089. Epub 2010 Jan 25.

143. Panzica GC, Viglietti-Panzica C, Mura E, et al. Effects of xenoestrogens on the differentiation of behaviorally-relevant neural circuits. *Front Neuroendocrinol*. 2007. 28(4):179–200. Epub 2007 Aug 6.

144. Nashev LG, Schuster D, Laggner C, et al. The UV-filter benzophenone-1 inhibits 17β-hydroxysteroid dehydrogenase type 3: Virtual screening as a strategy to identify potential endocrine disrupting chemicals. *Biochem Pharmcol*. 2010. 79(8):1189-1199. Epub 2009 Dec 11.

145. Schlumpf M, Schmid P, Durrer S, et. al. Endocrine activity and developmental toxicity of cosmetic UV filters–an update. *Toxicology*. 2004. 205:113–122.
    Goldstein JM, Seidman LJ, Horton NJ, et al. Normal sexual dimorphism of the adult human brain assessed by in vivo magnetic resonance imaging. Cereb Cortex. 2001. 11(6):490-497. Available at: www.cercor.oxfordjournals.org/content/11/6/490.full.

146. Rubin BS, Lenkowski JR, Schaeberle CM, Vandenberg LN, Ronsheim PM, Soto AM. Evidence of altered brain sexual differentiation in mice exposed perinatally to low, environmentally relevant levels of bisphenol A. *Endocrinology*. 2006. 147(8):3681-3691. Epub 2006 May 4.

147. Panzica GC, Viglietti-Panzica C, Ottinger MA. Introduction: neurobiological impact of environmental estrogens. *Brain Res Bull*. 2005. 65(3):187-191.

148. Ottinger MA, Lavoie E, Thompson N, et al. Neuroendocrine and behavioral effects of embryonic exposure to endocrine disrupting chemicals in birds. *Brain Res Rev*. 2008. 57(2):376-385. Epub 2007 Sep 19.

149. Ottinger MA, Lavoie ET, Thompson N, Bohannon M, Dean K, Quinn MJ Jr. Is the gonadotropin releasing hormone system vulnerable to endocrine disruption in birds? *Gen Comp Endocrinol*. 2009. 163(1-2):104-108. Epub 2009 May 18.

150. Panzica GC, Viglietti-Panzica C, Mura E, et al. Effects of xenoestrogens on the differentiation of behaviorally-relevant neural circuits. *Front Neuroendocrinol*. 2007. 28(4):179–200. Epub 2007 Aug 6.

151. Bernanke J, Köhler HR. The impact of environmental chemicals on wildlife vertebrates. *Rev Environ Contam Toxicol*. 2009. 198:1-47.

152. Carlsen E, Giwercman A, Keiding N, Skakkebaek NE. Evidence for decreasing quality of semen during past 50 years. *BMJ*. 1992. 305(6854):609-613.

153. Toppari J, Virtanen HE, Main KM, Skakkebaek NE. Cryptorchidism and hypospadias as a sign of testicular dysgenesis syndrome (TDS): environmental connection. *Birth Defects Res A Clin Mol Teratol*. 2010. 88(10):910-919.

154. Okeke AA, Osegbe DN. Prevalence and characteristics of cryptorchidism in a Nigerian district. *BJU Int*. 2001. 88(9):941-945.
    Williams L. Nigeria. Bradt Travel Guides: England. 2008.

155. eMedicine Website. Sumfest, JM, Kolon TF, Rukstalis DB. Cryptorchidism. Available at: http://emedicine.medscape.com/article/438378-overview#a0199. Accessed 11/30/10. Accessed June 7, 2011.

156. Boisen KA, Kaleva M, Main KM, et. al. Difference in prevalence of congenital cryptorchidism in infants between two Nordic countries. *Lancet*. 2004. 363:9417:1264-1269.

157. Yoshida R, Fukami M, Sasagawa I, Hasegawa T, Kamatani N, Ogata T. Association of cryptorchidism with a specific haplotype of the estrogen receptor alpha gene: implication for the susceptibility to estrogenic environmental endocrine disruptors. *J Clin Endocrinol Metab*. 2005. 90(8):4716-4721.

158. Toppari J, Haavisto AM, Alanen M. Changes in male reproductive health and effects of endocrine disruptors in Scandinavian countries. *Cad Saúde Pública*. 2002. 18(2):412-420. Epub 2002 Aug 16.

Virtanen HE, Toppari J. Epidemiology and pathogenesis of cryptorchidism. *Hum Reprod Update*. 2008. 14(1):49-58. Epub 2007 Nov 21.

159. Roberts J. Hypospadias surgery past, present and future. *Curr Opin Urol*. 2010. 20(6):483-489.

160. Porter MP, Faizan MK, Grady RW, Mueller BA. Hypospadias in Washington State: maternal risk factors and prevalence trends. *Pediatrics*. 2005. 115(4):e495-9. Epub 2005 Mar 1.

161. Carmichael SL, Shaw GM, Nelson V, Selvin S, Torfs CP, Curry CJ. Hypospadias in California: trends and descriptive epidemiology. *Epidemiology*. 2003. 14(6):701–706.

162. Carmichael SL, Shaw GM, Laurent C, Olney RS, Lammer EJ; National Birth Defects Prevention Study. Maternal reproductive and demographic characteristics as risk factors for (186.) Kojima Y, Kohri K, Hayashi Y. Genetic pathway of external genitalia formation and molecular etiology of hypospadias. *J Pediatr Urol*. 2010. 6(4):346-354. Epub 2009 Dec 7.

163. Kojima Y, Kohri K, Hayashi Y. Genetic pathway of external genitalia formation and molecular etiology of hypospadias. *J Pediatr Urol*. 2010. 6(4):346-354. Epub 2009 Dec 7.

Virtanen HE, Toppari J. Epidemiology and pathogenesis of cryptorchidism. *Hum Reprod Update*. 2008. 14(1):49-58. Epub 2007 Nov 21.

Main KM, Skakkebaek NE, Virtanen HE, Toppari J. Genital anomalies in boys and the environment. *Best Pract Res Clin Endocrinol Metab*. 2010. 24(2):270-289.

Toppari J, Virtanen HE, Main KM, Skakkebaek NE. Cryptorchidism and hypospadias as a sign of testicular dysgenesis syndrome (TDS): environmental connection. *Birth Defects Res A Clin Mol Teratol*. 2010. 88(10):910-¬919.

164. Carmichael SL, Herring AH, Sjödin A, et al. Hypospadias and halogenated organic pollutant levels in maternal mid-pregnancy serum samples. *Chemosphere*. 2010. 80(6):641-646. Epub 2010 May 21.

165. National Cancer Institute (USA) (USA) Website. Cancer Statistics: Testis. Available at: www.seer.cancer.gov/csr/1973_1999/testis.pdf. Accessed December 22, 2010.

166. Looijenga LH, Gillis AJ, Stoop HJ, Hersmus R, Oosterhuis JW. Chromosomes and expression in human testicular germ-cell tumors: insight into their cell of origin and pathogenesis. *Ann N Y Acad Sci*. 2007. 1120:187-214. Epub 2007 Oct 2.

167. Rajpert-de Meyts E, Hoei-Hansen CE. From gonocytes to testicular cancer: the role of impaired gonadal development. *Ann N Y Acad Sci*. 2007. 1120:168-180.

168. Myrup C, Westergaard T, Schnack T, et al. Testicular cancer risk in first- and second-generation immigrants to Denmark. *J Natl Cancer Inst*. 2008. 100(1):41-47. Epub 2007 Dec 25.

169. Joffe M. What has happened to human fertility? *Hum Reprod*. 2010. 25(2):295–307. Epub 2009 Nov 19.

170. Skakkebaek NE. Endocrine Disrupters and Testicular Dysgenesis Syndrome. *Horm Res*. 2002. 57(Suppl.2):43.

Urology Health Website. Glossary: testicular dysgenesis. Available at: www. urologyhealth.org. Accessed November 30, 2010.

171. Bansal AK, Bilaspuri GS. Impacts of oxidative stress and antioxidants on semen functions. Vet Med Int. 2010. pii: 686137

172. Sikka SC. Oxidative stress and role of antioxidants in normal and abnormal sperm function. *Front Biosci*. 1996. 1:e78-86.

173. Auger J, Kunstmann JM, Czyglik, F, Jouannet P. Decline in semen quality among fertile men in Paris during the past 20 years. *N Engl J Med*. 1995. 332(5):281-285.

174. European Science Foundation Website. Science Policy Briefing 40 – Male Reproductive Health: Its impacts in relation to general wellbeing and low European fertility rates – September 2010. Available at: www.esf.org/nc/ publications/medical-sciences/print.html?tx_ccdamdl_cart%5Badd%5D=2 7148&cHash=5f3aac48df. Accessed May 3, 2011.

175. European Science Foundation Website. Science Policy Briefing 40 – Male Reproductive Health: Its impacts in relation to general wellbeing and low European fertility rates – September 2010. Available at: www.esf.org/nc/ publications/medical-sciences/print.html?tx_ccdamdl_cart%5Badd%5D=2 7148&cHash=5f3aac48df. Accessed May 3, 2011.

Jensen TK, Jacobsen R, Christensen K, Nielsen NC, Bostofte E. Good semen quality and life expectancy: a cohort study of 43,277 men. *Am J Epidemiol*. 2009. 170(5):559-565. Epub 2009 Jul 27.

176. European Science Foundation Website. Science Policy Briefing 40 – Male Reproductive Health: Its impacts in relation to general wellbeing and low European fertility rates – September 2010. Available at: www.esf.org/nc/ publications/medical-sciences/print.html?tx_ccdamdl_cart%5Badd%5D=2 7148&cHash=5f3aac48df. Accessed May 3, 2011.

Internal Medicine News Website. Smith J. ESF sounds the alarm on male infertility. Available at: www.internalmedicinenews.com/news/nephrology-urology/single-article/esf-sounds-alarm-on-male-infertility/0f039485f0. html. Accessed December 23, 2010.

Andersen AG, Jensen TK, Carlsen E, et al. High frequency of suboptimal semen quality in an unselected population of young men. *Hum Reprod*. 2000. 15(2):366-372.

Jørgensen N, Carlsen E, Nermoen I, et al. East-West gradient in semen quality in the Nordic-Baltic area: a study of men from the general population in Denmark, Norway, Estonia and Finland. *Hum Reprod*. 2002. 17(8):2199-2208.

Skakkebaek NE, Rajpert-De Meyts E, Main KM. Testicular dysgenesis syndrome: an increasingly common developmental disorder with environmental aspects. *Hum Reprod*. 2001. 16(5):972-978.

Jensen TK, Jacobsen R, Christensen K, Nielsen NC, Bostofte E. Good semen quality and life expectancy: a cohort study of 43,277 men. *Am J Epidemiol*. 2009. 170(5):559-565. Epub 2009 Jul 27.

177. European Science Foundation Website. Science Policy Briefing 40 – Male Reproductive Health: Its impacts in relation to general wellbeing and low European fertility rates – September 2010. Available at: www.esf.org/nc/ publications/medical-sciences/print.html?tx_ccdamdl_cart%5Badd%5D=2 7148&cHash=5f3aac48df. Accessed May 3, 2011.

Jensen TK, Jacobsen R, Christensen K, Nielsen NC, Bostofte E. Good semen quality and life expectancy: a cohort study of 43,277 men. *Am J Epidemiol.* 2009. 170(5):559-565. Epub 2009 Jul 27.

178. Dr. Qaadri Website. Testosterone, Estrogen and Early Puberty. Available at: www.doctorq.ca/testosterone-estrogen-early-puberty.html. Accessed June 7, 2011.

179. Wolff MS, Teitelbaum SL, Windham G, et al. Pilot study of urinary biomarkers of phytoestrogens, phthalates, and phenols in girls. *Environ Health Perspect.* 2007. 115(1):116-121.

Zero Breast Cancer Website. Barlow J, Johnson JA. Breast Cancer and the Environment Research Centers: Early Life Exposure to Phenols and Breast Cancer Risk in Later Years. Fact Sheet on Phenols. Available at: www. zerobreastcancer.org/research/bcerc_factsheets_phenols.pdf. Accessed December 28, 2010.

180. WebMD Web site. Freeman D. Experts explain the causes and treatments of gynecomastia, or male breast enlargement. Available at: http://men.webmd. com/features/male-breast-enlargement-gynecomastia?page=2. Accessed December 22, 2010.

181. The Guardian Website. McVeigh K. Surgeons report surge in 'man boob' operations. Available at: www.guardian.co.uk/lifeandstyle/2010/jan/31/ surgeons-surge-man-boob-operations. Accessed June 17, 2011.

British Association of Aesthetic Plastic Surgeons Web site. Britons over the moob: male breast reduction nearly doubles in 2009. Available at: www. baaps.org.uk/about-us/press-releases/584-britons-over-the-moob-male-breast-reduction-nearly-doubles-in-2009. Accessed December 13, 2010.

182. ISAPS Web site. ISAPS International Survey on Aesthetic/Cosmetic Procedures Performed in 2009. Available at: www.isaps.org/stats.php. Accessed December 13, 2010.

[Note for United States numbers: Whereas this study focused exclusively on board-certified Plastic Surgeons, surveys conducted by the American Society of Aesthetic Plastic Surgery include board-certified Plastic Surgeons as well as board-certified Dermatologists and board-certified Otolaryngologists (ears, nose and throat specialists).]

183. Zero Breast Cancer Website. Barlow J, Johnson JA. Breast Cancer and the Environment Research Centers: Early Life Exposure to Phenols and Breast Cancer Risk in Later Years. Fact Sheet on Phenols. Available at: www. zerobreastcancer.org/research/bcerc_factsheets_phenols.pdf. Accessed December 28, 2010.

Vandenberg LN, Maffini MV, Wadia PR, Sonnenschein C, Rubin BS, Soto AM. Exposure to environmentally relevant doses of the xenoestrogen bisphenol-A alters development of the fetal mouse mammary gland. *Endocrinology.* 2007. 148(1):116-127. Epub 2006 Oct 5.

Durando M, Kass L, Piva J, Sonnenschein C, Soto AM, Munoz-de-Toro M. Prenatal bisphenol A exposure induces preneoplastic lesions in the mammary gland in Wistar rats. *Environ Health Perspect.* 2007. 115(1):80-86.

184. Schlumpf M, Cotton B, Conscience M, Haller V, Steinmann B, Lichtensteiger W. In vitro and in vivo estrogenicity of UV screens. *Environ Health Perspect.* 2001. 109(3):239–244.

Schlumpf M, Schmid P, Durrer S, et. al. Endocrine activity and developmental toxicity of cosmetic UV filters–an update. *Toxicology.* 2004. 205:113–122.

185. WebMD Website. Hitti M. FDA OKs New Sunscreen: Anthelios SX Includes Active Ingredient Previously Unmarketed in U.S. Available at: www.webmd.com/news/20060724/fda-oks-sunscreen. Accessed April 27, 2011.

186. Klinubol P, Asawanonda P, Wanichwecharungruang SP. Transdermal penetration of UV filters. *Skin Pharmacol Physiol.* 2008. 21(1):23-29. Epub 2007 Oct 2.

187. Armeni T, Damiani E, Battino M, Greci L, Principato G. Lack of in vitro protection by a common sunscreen ingredient on UVA-induced cytotoxicity in keratinocytes. *Toxicology.* 2004. 203(1-3):165-178.

188. Nakagawa Y, Suzuki T. Metabolism of 2-hydroxy-4-methoxybenzophenone in isolated rat hepatocytes and xenoestrogenic effects of its metabolites on MCF-7 human breast cancer cells. *Chem Bio Interact.* 2002. 139(2):115–128.

189. Ziolkowska A, Rucinski M, Pucher A, Tortorella C, Nussdorfer GG, Malendowicz LK. Expression of osteoblast marker genes in rat calvarial osteoblast-like cells, and effects of the endocrine disrupters diphenylolpropane, benzophenone-3, resveratrol and silymarin. *Chem Biol Interact.* 2006. 164(3):147-156. Epub 2006 Oct 1.

190. Schmutzler C, Bacinski A, Gotthardt I, et. al. The ultraviolet filter benzophenone 2 interferes with the thyroid hormone axis in rats and is a potent in vitro inhibitor of human recombinant thyroid peroxidase. *Endocrinology.* 2007. 148(6):2835-2844. Epub 2007 Mar 22.

Crofton KM. Thyroid disrupting chemicals: mechanisms and mixtures. *Int J Androl.* 2008. 31(2):209-223. Epub 2008 Jan 22.

Capen CC. Mechanistic data and risk assessment of selected toxic end points of the thyroid gland. *Toxicol Pathol.* 1997. 25(1):39–48.

Boas M, Feldt-Rasmussen U, Skakkebaek NE, Main KM. Environmental chemicals and thyroid function. *Eur J Endocrinol.* 2006. 154(5):599-611.

Miller MD, Crofton KM, Rice DC, Zoeller RT. Thyroid-disrupting chemicals: interpreting upstream biomarkers of adverse outcomes. *Environ Health Perspect.* 2009. 117(7):1033–1041. Epub 2009 Feb 12.

Crofton KM, Craft ES, Hedge JM, et al. Thyroid-hormone-disrupting chemicals: evidence for dose- dependent additivity or synergism. *Environ Health Perspect.* 2005. 113(11):1549-1554.

191. Klammer H, Schlecht C, Wuttke W, et al. Effects of a 5-day treatment with the UV-filter octyl-methoxycinnamate (OMC) on the function of the hypothalamo-pituitary-thyroid function in rats. *Toxicology.* 2007. 238(2-3):192-199. Epub 2007 Jun 23.

192. Zoeller TR, Dowling AL, Herzig CT, Iannacone EA, Gauger KJ, Bansal R. Thyroid hormone, brain development, and the environment. *Environ Health Perspect.* 2002. 110(Suppl 3):355-361.

Jugan ML, Levi Y, Blondeau JP. Endocrine disruptors and thyroid hormone physiology. *Biochem Pharmacol.* 2010. 79(7):939-947. Epub 2009 Nov 12.

193. Wisconsin Medical Society Website. Treffert DA. Autistic Disorder: 52 Years Later: Some Common Sense Conclusions. Available at: www.wisconsinmedicalsociety.org/savant_syndrome/savant_articles/autistic_disorder. Accessed June 7, 2011.

Rice C. Prevalence of Autism Spectrum Disorders–Autism and Developmental Disabilities Monitoring Network, United States, 2006. CDC MMWR. December 18, 2009 / 58(SS10);1-20. Available at: www.cdc.gov/mmwr/preview/mmwrhtml/ss5810a1.htm.

194. Autism Speaks Website. Autism speaks responds to new pediatrics autism study putting prevalence at 1 in 91 American children, including 1 in 58 boys. Available at: www.autismspeaks.org/press/autism_nchs_prevalence_study_1_in_91.php. Accessed June 17, 2011.

195. Wisconsin Medical Society Website. Treffert DA. Autistic Disorder: 52 Years Later: Some Common Sense Conclusions. Available at: www.wisconsinmedicalsociety.org/savant_syndrome/savant_articles/autistic_disorder. Accessed June 7, 2011

    Age of Autism Website. Olmsted D. Olmsted on Autism: 1 in 10,000 Amish. Available at: www.ageofautism.com/2009/04/olmsted-on-autism-1-in-10000-amish.html. Accessed April 27, 2011.

196. Wisconsin Medical Society Website. Treffert DA. Autistic Disorder: 52 Years Later: Some Common Sense Conclusions. Available at: www.wisconsinmedicalsociety.org/savant_syndrome/savant_articles/autistic_disorder. Accessed June 7, 2011.

197. Jones RM, Wheelwright S, Farrell K, et al. Brief report: female-to-male transsexual people and autistic traits. *J Autism Dev Disord.* 2011 Mar 30. [Epub ahead of print].

198. Colborn T. Neurodevelopment and endocrine disruption. *Environ Health Perspect.* 2004. 112(9):944-949.

199. Porterfield SP. Vulnerability of the developing brain to thyroid abnormalities: environmental insults to the thyroid system. *Environ Health Perspect.* 1994. 102(Suppl 2):125-130.

200. Sadamatsu M, Kanai H, Xu X, Liu Y, Kato N. Review of animal models for autism: implication of thyroid hormone. *Congenit Anom* (Kyoto). 2006. 46(1):1-9.

    Román GC. Autism: transient in utero hypothyroxinemia related to maternal flavonoid ingestion during pregnancy and to other environmental antithyroid agents. *J Neurol Sci.* 2007. 262(1-2):15-26. Epub 2007 Jul 24.

201. Adams JB, Holloway CE, George F, Quig D. Analyses of toxic metals and essential minerals in the hair of Arizona children with autism and associated conditions, and their mothers. *Biol Trace Elem Res.* 2006. 110(3):193-209.

202. Kajta M, Wójtowicz A. Neurodevelopmental disorders in response to hormonally active environmental pollutants. *Przegl Lek.* 2010. 67(11):1194-1199.

203. Mandell DS, Wiggins LD, Carpenter LA, et. al. Racial/ethnic disparities in the identification of children with autism spectrum disorders. *Am J Public Health.* 2009. 99(3):493-498. Epub 2008 Dec 23.

204. Heindel JJ. Animal models for probing the developmental basis of disease and dysfunction paradigm. *Basic Clin Pharmacol Toxicol.* 2008. 102(2):76-81.

205. Heindel JJ, vom Saal FS. Role of nutrition and environmental endocrine disrupting chemicals during the perinatal period on the aetiology of obesity. *Mol Cell Endocrinol.* 2009. 304(1-2): 90–96. Epub 2009 Mar 9.

206. Newbold RR. Impact of environmental endocrine disrupting chemicals on the development of obesity. *Hormones* (Athens). 2010. 9(3):206-217.

207. Kortenkamp A. Low dose mixture effects of endocrine disrupters: implications for risk assessment and epidemiology. *Int J Androl.* 2008. 31(2):233-240. Epub 2008 Jan 29.

208. Ocean World Web site. Coral Reef Destruction and Conservation. Available at: www.oceanworld.tamu.edu/students/coral/coral5.htm. Accessed December 14, 2010.

209. Cook-Anderson G. Recent Coral Bleaching at Great Barrier Reef. NASA Goddard Space Flight Center. 2006. Available at: http://news.mongabay. com/2006/0405-nasa.html. Accessed January 24, 2011.

210. Bright Hub Web site. Scott W. Average ocean temperature increases 1996 to 2010. Available at: www.brighthub.com/engineering/marine/articles/81834.aspx. Accessed December 14, 2010.

211. NOAA National Climate Data Center Website. State of the Climate: Global Analysis for December 2009. Available at: www.ncdc.noaa.gov/sotc/ global/2009/12. Accessed June 9, 2011.

212. Summit County Citizens Voice Website. Berwyn B. Forida's coral reefs hit hard by record cold water temps. Available at: http://summitcountyvoice. com/2011/04/12/floridas-coral-reefs-hit-hard-by-

213. Cook-Anderson G. Recent Coral Bleaching at Great Barrier Reef. NASA Goddard Space Flight Center. 2006. Available at: http://news.mongabay. com/2006/0405-nasa.html. Accessed January 24, 2011.

214. Seaworld Web site. Corals and coral reefs: longevity and causes of death. Available at: www.seaworld.org/animal-info/info-books/coral/longevity. htm. Accessed December 14, 2010.

215. Rasher DB, Hay ME. Chemically rich seaweeds poison corals when not controlled by herbivores. Proc Natl Acad Sci USA. 2010. 107(21):9683-9688.

216. Wooldridge SA. Water quality and coral bleaching thresholds: Formalising the linkage for the inshore reefs of the Great Barrier Reef, Australia. Mar Pollut Bull. 2009. 58(5):745-751. Epub 2009 Feb 23.

217. eMedicine Website. Ho H, Do TH, Ho TT. Vibrio Infections. www.emedicine. medscape.com/article/232038-overview. Accessed February 5, 2011.

218. Alves N, Oswaldo S, Neto M. Diversity and pathogenic potential of vibrios isolated from Abrolhos Bank corals. Special Issue: Vibrio Ecology. 2010. 2(1):90–95. Available at: http://onlinelibrary.wiley.com/doi/10.1111/ j.1758-2229.2009.00101.x/full. Accessed May 3, 2011.

219. Rosenberg E, Falkowitz L. The Vibrio shiloi/Oculina patagonica model system of coral bleaching. Annu Rev Microbiol. 2004. 58:143–159.
Banin E, Khare SK, Naider F, Rosenberg E. A proline-rich peptide from the coral pathogen Vibrio shiloi that inhibits photosynthesis of zooxanthellae. Appl Environ Microbiol. 2001. 67(4):1536–1541.

220. Ben-Haim Y, Banim E, Kushmaro A, Loya Y, Rosenberg E. Inhibition of photosynthesis and bleaching of zooxanthellae by the coral pathogen: Vibrio shiloi. Environ Microbiol. 1999. 1(3):223-229.
Banin E, Khare SK, Naider F, Rosenberg E. A proline-rich peptide from the coral pathogen Vibrio shiloi that inhibits photosynthesis of zooxanthellae. Appl Environ Microbiol. 2001. 67(4):1536–1541.

221. Banin E, Israely T, Fine M, Loya Y, Rosenberg E. Role of endosymbiotic zooxanthellae and coral mucus in the adhesion of the coral-bleaching pathogen Vibrio shiloi to its host. FEMS Microbiol Lett. 2001. 199(1):33–37.

222. Williams GJ, Knapp IS, Maragos JE, Davy SK. Modeling patterns of coral bleaching at a remote Central Pacific atoll. Mar Pollut Bull. 2010. 60(9):1467–1476. Epub 2010 Jun 11.

223. Bourne D, Iida1 Y, Uthicke1 S, Smith-Keune1 C. Changes in coral-associated microbial communities during a bleaching event. ISME J. 2008. 2(4):350–363. Epub 2008 Dec 6.

224. Australian Government Website. Past bleaching events on the Great Barrier Reef. Available at: www.aims.gov.au/docs/research/climate-change/coral-bleaching/bleaching-events.html. Accessed June 17, 2011.

Day J. Marine park management and monitoring: lessons for adaptive management from the Great Barrier Reef. In: Managing protected areas in a changing world: proceedings of the Fourth International Conference on Science and Management of Protected Areas,14-19 May 2000. Science & Management of Protected Areas Assoc. 2002. 1258-1282. Available at: http://ioc3.unesco.org/marinesp/files/Adaptive%20management%20 SAMPA.pdf. Accessed December 14, 2010.

225. Barrier Reef Australia Website. Great Barrier Reef. Available at: www. barrierreefaustralia.com/the-great-barrier-reef/great-barrier-reef-info.htm. Accessed July 6, 2011.

226. Cook-Anderson G. Recent Coral Bleaching at Great Barrier Reef. NASA Goddard Space Flight Center. 2006. Available at: http://news.mongabay. com/2006/0405-nasa.html. Accessed January 24, 2011.

227. Australian Government Website. Tourist visit to the entire Great Barrier Reef Marine Park. Available at: www.gbrmpa.gov.au/corp_site/key_issues/ tourism/management/gbr_visitation/numbers/reef_wide. Accessed June 20, 2011.

228. Danovaro R, Bongiorni L, Corinaldesi C, et al. Sunscreens cause coral bleaching by promoting viral infections. *Environ Health Perspect.* 2008. 116(4):441–447.

229. Belize Tourism Web Site. The beginnings of tourism in Belize. Available at: www. belizetourism.org/belize-tourism/history.html. Accessed October 25, 2010.

Belize Tourism Website. The beginnings of tourism in Belize. Available at: http://belizedev.com/belizetourism/content/view/129/178/. Accessed June 19, 2011.

USA Today Web site: Bly L. Belize's coral reef is gorgeous but threatened. Available at: www.usatoday.com/travel/news/environment/2008-03-13-belize_N.htm. Accessed October 25, 2010.

Brown BE. Coral bleaching: causes and consequences. *Coral Reefs.* 1997. 16(Suppl):S129–S138.

230. Ainsworth TD, Fine M, Roff G, Hoegh-Guldberg O. Bacteria are not the primary cause of bleaching in the Mediterranean coral Oculina patagonica. *ISME J.* 2008. 2(1):67–73. Epub 2007 Dec 6.

231. Juhasz A, Ho E, Bender E, Fong F. Does use of tropical beaches by tourists and island residents result in damage to fringing coral reefs? A case study in Moorea French Polynesia. *Mar Pollut Bull.* 2010. 60(12):2251–2256. Epub 2010 Sep 15.

232. Danovaro R, Bongiorni L, Corinaldesi C, et al. Sunscreens cause coral bleaching by promoting viral infections. *Environ Health Perspect.* 2008. 116(4):441–447.

233. Science Daily Website. Nanoparticles Delivering Drugs Can Kill Skin, Breast Cancer Cells. Available at: www.sciencedaily.com/releases/2008/12/081215151147. htm. Accessed May 9, 2011.

234. Nowack B, Bucheli TD. Occurrence, behavior and effects of nanoparticles in the environment. Environ Pollut. 2007. 150(1):5-22.

235. Farré M, Gajda-Schrantz K, Kantiani L, Barceló D. Ecotoxicity and analysis of nanomaterials in the aquatic environment. *Anal Bioanal Chem.* 2009. 393(1):81-95. Epub 2008 Nov 6.

236. Li JJ, Muralikrishnan S, Ng CT, Yung LY, Bay BH. Nanoparticle-induced pulmonary toxicity. *Exp Biol Med* (Maywood). 2010. 235(9):1025-1033. Epub 2010 Aug 18.

237. Landsiedel R, Ma-Hock L, Van Ravenzwaay B, et al. Gene toxicity studies on titanium dioxide and zinc oxide nanomaterials used for UV-protection in cosmetic formulations. *Nanotoxicology*. 2010. 4:364-381.

238. New Orleans Web site. Human-Environment Interactions: Understanding Change in Dynamic Systems: Post meeting info: abstract book download. Available at: http://neworleans.setac.org/sites/default/files/abstract%20 book.pdf. Accessed December 22, 2010.
    Zhang J, Wages M. Effect of titanium dioxides nanomaterials and ultraviolet light coexposure on xenopus laevis. SP014 In: SETAC North America 30th Annual Meeting. 2010. New Orleans, LA. USA. Available at: http:// neworleans.setac.org/sites/default/files/abstract%20book.pdf. Accessed December 22, 2010.

239. Moore MN. Do nanoparticles present ecotoxicological risks for the health of the aquatic environment? *Environ Int*. 2006. 32(8):967-976. Epub 2006 Jul 21.

240. Clearwater SJ, Farag AM, Meyer JS. Review: Bioavailability and toxicity of dietborne copper and zinc to fish. *Comp Biochem Physiol C Toxicol Pharmacol*. 2002. 132(3):269–313.

241. Mortimer M, Kasemets K, Kahru A. Toxicity of ZnO and CuO nanoparticles to ciliated protozoa Tetrahymena thermophila. *Toxicology*. 2010. 269(2-3):182–189. Epub 2009 Jul 19.

242. Baun A, Hartmann NB, Grieger K, Kusk KO. Ecotoxicity of engineered nanoparticles to aquatic invertebrates: a brief review and recommendations for future toxicity testing. *Ecotoxicology*. 2008. 17(5):387-395. Epub 2008 Apr 19.

243. Ju-Nam Y, Lead JR. Manufactured nanoparticles: an overview of their chemistry, interactions and potential environmental implications. *Sci Total Environ*. 2008. 400(1-3):396-414. Epub 2008 Aug 19.

244. Zhu X, Chang Y, Chen Y. Toxicity and bioaccumulation of TiO2 nanoparticle aggregates in Daphnia magna. *Chemosphere*. 2010. 78(3):209-215. Epub 2009 Dec 5.

245. Hao L, Wang Z, Xing B. Effect of sub-acute exposure to TiO2 nanoparticles on oxidative stress and histopathological changes in Juvenile Carp (Cyprinus carpio). *J Environ Sci* (China). 2009. 21(10):1459-1466.

246. Gamer AO, Leibold E, van Ravenzwaay B. The in vitro absorption of microfine zinc oxide and titanium dioxide through porcine skin. *Toxicology in Vitro*. 2006. 20(3):301–307. Epub 2005 Sep 21.

247. Schilling K, Bradford B, Castelli D, et al. Human safety review of "nano" titanium dioxide and zinc oxide. *Photochem Photobiol*. 2010. 9(4):495-509.

248. Sohn FS, Cohen JB. Do no harm: nanotechnology and sunscreens. *Clin Exp Dermatol*. 2008. 33(6):776.

249. Gulson B, McCall M, Korsch M, et al. Small amounts of zinc from zinc oxide particles in sunscreens applied outdoors are absorbed through human skin. *Toxicological Science*. 2010.118(1):140-149.

250. Senzui M, Tamura T, Miura K, Ikarashi Y, Watanabe Y, Fujii M. Study on penetration of titanium dioxide (TiO(2)) nanoparticles into intact and damaged skin in vitro. *J Toxicol Sci*. 2010. 35(1):107-113.

251. Kobo Products Inc. Website. Nguyen U, Scholossman D. Stability Study of Avobenzone with Inorganic Sunscreens. Available at: www.koboproductsinc. com/Downloads/NYSCC-Avobenzone.pdf. Accessed March 20, 2011.

252. Rossi EM, Pylkkänen L, Koivisto AJ, Airway exposure to silica-coated TiO$_2$ nanoparticles induces pulmonary neutrophilia in mice. *Toxicol Sci.* 2010. 113(2):422-433. Epub 2009 Oct 29.

253. Wu J, Liu W, Xue C, et al. Toxicity and penetration of TiO$_2$ nanoparticles in hairless mice and porcine skin after subchronic dermal exposure. *Toxicol Lett.* 2009. 191(1):1-8. Epub 2009 Jan 6.

254. Dunford R, Salinaro A, Cai L, et al. Chemical oxidation and DNA damage catalysed by inorganic sunscreen ingredients. *FEBS Lett.* 1997. 418(1-2):87–90.

255. Nel A, Xia T, Mädler L, Li N. Toxic potential of materials at the nanolevel. *Science.* 2006. 311(5761):622-627.

256. Pan Z, Lee W, Slutsky L, Clark RA, Pernodet N, Rafailovich MH. Adverse effects of titanium dioxide nanoparticles on human dermal fibroblasts and how to protect cells. *Small.* 2009. 5(4):511-520.

257. Rossi EM, Pylkkänen L, Koivisto AJ, Airway exposure to silica-coated TiO$_2$ nanoparticles induces pulmonary neutrophilia in mice. *Toxicol Sci.* 2010. 113(2):422-433. Epub 2009 Oct 29.

258. Shukla RK, Sharma V, Pandey AK, Singh S, Sultana S, Dhawan A. ROS-mediated genotoxicity induced by titanium dioxide nanoparticles in human epidermal cells. *Toxicol in Vitro.* 2011. 25(1):231-241. Epub 2010 Nov 17. [Epub ahead of print] doi: 10.1016/j.tiv.2010.11.008.

259. Baer DR, Gaspar D J, Nachimuthu P, Techane SD, Castner DG. 2010. Application of surface chemical analysis tools for characterization of nanoparticles. *Anal Bioanal Chem.* 2010. 396:983-1002. Epub 2010 Jan 6.

Dhawan A, Sharma V. 2010. Toxicity assessment of nanomaterials: methods and challenges. *Anal Bioanal Chem.* 2010. 398(2):589-605. Epub 2010 Jul 22.

Doak SH, Griffiths SM, Manshian B, et al. 2009. Confounding experimental considerations in nanogenotoxicology. *Mutagenesis.* 2009. 24(4):285-293. Epub 2009 Apr 7.

Monteiro-Riviere NA, Inman AO, Zhang LW. 2009. Limitations and relative utility of screening assays to assess engineered nanoparticle toxicity in a human cell line. *Toxicol Appl Pharmacol.* 2009. 234(2):222-235. Epub 2008 Oct 17.

Stone V, Johnston H, Schins RP. Development of in vitro systems for nanotoxicology: methodological considerations. *Crit Rev Toxicol.* 2009. 39(7):613-626.

260. Shukla RK, Sharma V, Pandey AK, Singh S, Sultana S, Dhawan A. ROS-mediated genotoxicity induced by titanium dioxide nanoparticles in human epidermal cells. *Toxicol in Vitro.* 2011. 25(1):231-241. Epub 2010 Nov 17. [Epub ahead of print] doi: 10.1016/j.tiv.2010.11.008.

261. National Toxicology Program Web site. Descriptions of NTP study types: micronucleus. Available at: www.ntp.niehs.nih.gov/?objectid=16D65516-BA99-8D3E-BEFF712372F4B675. Accessed November 24, 2010.

262. Shukla RK, Sharma V, Pandey AK, Singh S, Sultana S, Dhawan A. ROS-mediated genotoxicity induced by titanium dioxide nanoparticles in human epidermal cells. *Toxicol in Vitro.* 2011. 25(1):231-241. Epub 2010 Nov 17. [Epub ahead of print] doi: 10.1016/j.tiv.2010.11.008.

263. Li Y, Li J, Yin J, et al. Systematic influence induced by 3 nm titanium dioxide following intratracheal instillation of mice. *J Nanosci Nanotechnol.* 2010. 10(12):8544-8549.

264. Wu J, Liu W, Xue C, et al. Toxicity and penetration of TiO_2 nanoparticles in hairless mice and porcine skin after subchronic dermal exposure. *Toxicol Lett.* 2009. 191(1):1-8. Epub 2009 Jan 6.

265. Wang Z, Zhang K, Zhao J, Liu X, Xing B. Adsorption and inhibition of butyrylcholinesterase by different engineered nanoparticles. *Chemosphere.* 2010. 79(1):86-92. Epub 2010 Jan 20.

266. Liu S, Xu L, Zhang T, Ren G, Yang Z. Oxidative stress and apoptosis induced by nanosized titanium dioxide in PC12 cells. *Toxicology.* 2010. 267(1-3):172-177. Epub 2009 Nov 14.

267. Science Daily Website. Nanoparticles Used in Common Household Items Cause Genetic Damage in Mice. Available at: www.sciencedaily.com/releases/2009/11/091116165739.htm. Accessed June 17, 2011. Interview of co-author of: Trouiller B, Reliene R, Westbrook A, Solaimani P, Schiestl RH. Titanium dioxide nanoparticles induce DNA damage and genetic instability in vivo in mice. *Cancer Res.* 2009. 69(22):8784-8789. Epub 2009 Nov 3.

268. Trouiller B, Reliene R, Westbrook A, Solaimani P, Schiestl RH. Titanium dioxide nanoparticles induce DNA damage and genetic instability in vivo in mice. *Cancer Res.* 2009. 69(22):8784–8789. Epub 2009 Nov 3.

269. Science Daily Website. Nanoparticles Used in Common Household Items Cause Genetic Damage in Mice. Available at: www.sciencedaily.com/releases/2009/11/091116165739.htm. Accessed June 17, 2011. Interview of co-author of: Trouiller B, Reliene R, Westbrook A, Solaimani P, Schiestl RH. Titanium dioxide nanoparticles induce DNA damage and genetic instability in vivo in mice. *Cancer Res.* 2009. 69(22):8784-8789. Epub 2009 Nov 3.

270. Li JJ, Muralikrishnan S, Ng CT, Yung LY, Bay BH. Nanoparticle-induced pulmonary toxicity. *Exp Biol Med* (Maywood). 2010. 235(9):1025-1033. Epub 2010 Aug 18.

271. Chen HW, Su SF, Chien CT, et al. Titanium dioxide nanoparticles induce emphysema-like lung injury in mice. *FASEB J.* 2006. 20(13):2393-2395. Epub 2006 Oct 5.

272. Suite101 Website. Rorem S. Sea Creatures 101: Plankton: Teens of the Sea. Available at: www.suite101.com/article.cfm/aquatic_animals/65951. Accessed March 9, 2011.

Marinebio Website. Ocean Resources. Available at: www.marinebio.org/oceans/ocean-resources.asp. Accessed March 9, 2011.

Red Orbit Website. Phytoplankton decline seen over the last century. Available at: www.redorbit.com/news/science/1898198/phytoplankton_decline_seen_over_the_last_century/. Accessed November 27, 2010.

National Geographic Website. Source of half earth's oxygen gets little credit. Available at: http://news.nationalgeographic.com/news/2004/06/0607_040607_phytoplankton_2.html. Accessed December 23, 2010.

273. The Free Dictionary Website. Medical dictionary: zinc chloride. Available at: www.medical-dictionary.thefreedictionary.com/zinc+chloride. Accessed December 21, 2010.

Oregon State Univ. Website. Micronutrient information center: zinc. Available at: http://lpi.oregonstate.edu/infocenter/minerals/zinc/. Accessed December 23, 2010.

274. Miao AJ, Zhang XY, Luo Z, et al. Zinc oxide-engineered nanoparticles: dissolution and toxicity to marine phytoplankton. *Environ Toxicol Chem.* 2010. 29(12):2814-22. Epub 2010 Oct 7.

275. Answers.com Website. Phytoplankton. Available at: www.answers.com/topic/phytoplankton. Accessed November 27, 2010.

NASA Website. What are phytoplankton? Available at: www.earthobservatory. nasa.gov/Features/Phytoplankton/. Accessed December 22, 2010.

Miller RJ, Lenihan HS, Muller EB, Tseng N, Hanna SK, Keller AA. Impacts of metal oxide nanoparticles on marine phytoplankton. *Environ Sci Technol.* 2010. 44(19):7329-7334

276. Miller RJ, Lenihan HS, Muller EB, Tseng N, Hanna SK, Keller AA. Impacts of metal oxide nanoparticles on marine phytoplankton. *Environ Sci Technol.* 2010. 44(19):7329-7344.

277. Wong SW, Leung PT, Djurisić AB, Leung KM. Toxicities of nano zinc oxide to five marine organisms: influences of aggregate size and ion solubility. *Anal Bioanal Chem.* 2010. 396(2):609-618. Epub 2009 Nov 10.

278. Kahru A, Dubourguier HC. From ecotoxicology to nanoecotoxicology. *Toxicology.* 2010. 269(2-3):105-119. Epub 2009 Sep 2.

279. Ward JE, Kach DJ. Marine aggregates facilitate ingestion of nanoparticles by suspension-feeding bivalves. *Mar Environ Res.* 2009. 68(3):137-142. Epub 2009 May 24.

280. Adams LK, Lyon DY, Alvarez PJ. Comparative eco-toxicity of nanoscale TiO_2, $SiO2$, and ZnO water suspensions. *Water Res.* 2006. 0(19):3527-3532. Epub 2006 Sep 29.

281. Hodges ND, Moss SH, Davies DJ. Evidence for increased genetic damage due to the presence of a sunscreen agent, para-aminobenzoic acid, during irradiation with near ultraviolet light [proceedings]. *J Pharm Pharmacol.* 1976. 28 Suppl:53P.

Osgood PJ, Moss SH, Davies DJ. The sensitization of near-ultraviolet radiation killing of mammalian cells by the sunscreen agent para-aminobenzoic acid. *J Invest Dermatol.* 1982. 79(6):354-357.

Hodges ND, Moss SH, Davies DJ. Elucidation of the nature of genetic damage formed in the presence of the sunscreening agent, para-amino benzoic acid, during irradiation with near ultraviolet light [proceedings]. *J Pharm Pharmacol.* 1977. 29 Suppl:72P.

282. Matts PJ, Fink B. Chronic sun damage and the perception of age, health and attractiveness. *Photochem Photobiol Sci.* 2010. 9(4):421-431.

283. Schieke SM, Schroeder P, Krutmann J. Cutaneous effects of infrared radiation: from clinical observations to molecular response mechanisms. *Photodermatol Photoimmunol Photomed.* 2003. 19(5):228-234.

Agache PG, Humbert P, Maibach HI. *Measuring the Skin.* 1st ed. Springer. 2011.

284. Bachem A, Reed CI. The penetration of radiation through human skin. Am J Physiol. 1931. 97: 86–91. Cited in Schieke SM, Schroeder P, Krutmann J. Cutaneous effects of infrared radiation: from clinical observations to molecular response mechanisms. *Photodermatol Photoimmunol Photomed.* 2003. 19(5):228-234. Cited in Schieke SM, Schroeder P, Krutmann J. Cutaneous effects of infrared radiation: from clinical observations to molecular response mechanisms. *Photodermatol Photoimmunol Photomed.* 2003 Oct;19(5):228-34.

285. Schwartz RA. Infrared radiation as a carcinogenic agent. *Br J Dermatol*. 1978. 99(4):460-461.
286. Piazena H, Kelleher DK. Effects of infrared-A irradiation on skin: discrepancies in published data highlight the need for an exact consideration of physical and photobiological laws and appropriate experimental settings. *Photochem Photobiol*. 2010. 86(3):687-705. Epub 2010 Apr 16.
287. Kligman LH. Intensification of ultraviolet-induced dermal damage by infrared radiation. *Arch Dermatol Res*. 1982. 272(3-4):229-238.
288. Loggie BW, Eddy JA. Solar considerations in the development of cutaneous melanoma. *Semin Oncol*. 1988. 15(6):494-499.
289. Schieke SM, Schroeder P, Krutmann J. Cutaneous effects of infrared radiation: from clinical observations to molecular response mechanisms. *Photodermatol Photoimmunol Photomed*. 2003. 19(5):228-234.
290. Schroeder P, Calles C, Benesova T, Macaluso F, Krutmann J. Photoprotection beyond ultraviolet radiation–effective sun protection has to include protection against infrared A radiation-induced skin damage. *Skin Pharmacol Physiol*. 2010. 23(1):15-17. Epub 2010 Jan 14.
291. Kligman LH. Full spectrum solar radiation as a cause of dermal photodamage: UVB to infrared. *Acta Derm Venereol Suppl* (Stockh). 1987. 134:53-61.
292. Kim MS, Kim YK, Cho KH, Chung JH. Regulation of type I procollagen and MMP-1 expression after single or repeated exposure to infrared radiation in human skin. *Mech Ageing Dev*. 2006. 127(12):875-882. Epub 2006 Oct 25.
293. Kim HH, Lee MJ, Lee SR, et al. Augmentation of UV-induced skin wrinkling by infrared irradiation in hairless mice. *Mech Ageing Dev*. 2005. 126(11):1170-1177.
294. Cho S, Shin MH, Kim YK, et al. Effects of infrared radiation and heat on human skin aging in vivo. *J Investig Dermatol Symp Proc*. 2009. 14(1):15-19. doi:10.1038/jidsymp.2009.7.
295. Springer Images Website. Available at: www.springerimages.com/Images/MedicineAndPublicHealth/1-10.1007_978-3-540-89656-2_42-1. Accessed March 18, 2011.
    Schroeder P, Haendeler J, Krutmann J. The role of near infrared radiation in photoaging of the skin. *Exp Gerontol*. 2008. 43(7):629-632. Epub 2008 Apr 27.
    Bachem A, Reed CI. The penetration of radiation through human skin. *Am J Physiol*. 1931. 97:86–91. Cited in Schieke SM, Schroeder P, Krutmann J. Cutaneous effects of infrared radiation: from clinical observations to molecular response mechanisms. *Photodermatol Photoimmunol Photomed*. 2003. 19(5):228-234.
296. Skin Biology Website. The Biology of Skin and Aging Damage. Available at: www.skinbiology.com/skinhealth&aging.htm. Accessed March 19, 2011.
    Rijken F, Bruijnzeel PL. The pathogenesis of photoaging: the role of neutrophils and neutrophil-derived enzymes. *J Investig Dermatol Symp Proc*. 2009. 14(1):67-72.
297. Rijken F, Bruijnzeel PL. The pathogenesis of photoaging: the role of neutrophils and neutrophil-derived enzymes. *J Investig Dermatol Symp Proc*. 2009. 14(1):67-72.
298. Frank S, Oliver L, Lebreton-De Coster C, et al. Infrared radiation affects the mitochondrial pathway of apoptosis in human fibroblasts. *J Invest Dermatol*. 2004. 123(5):823-831.

Schroeder P, Calles C, Krutmann J. Prevention of infrared-A radiation mediated detrimental effects in human skin. *Skin Therapy Lett*. 2009. 14(5):4-5. Available at: www.skintherapyletter.com/2009/14.5/2.html. Accessed March 19, 2011.

Schroeder P, Lademann J, Darvin ME, et al. Infrared radiation-induced matrix metalloproteinase in human skin: implications for protection. *J Invest Dermatol*. 2008. 128(10): 2491–2497. Epub 2008 May 1.

299. Snow BJ, Rolfe FL, Lockhart MM, et al. A double-blind, placebo-controlled study to assess the mitochondria-targeted antioxidant MitoQ as a disease-modifying therapy in Parkinson's disease. *Mov Disord*. 2010. 25(11):1670-1674.

300. Schroeder P, Haendeler J, Krutmann J. The role of near infrared radiation in photoaging of the skin. *Exp Gerontol*. 2008. 43(7):629-632. Epub 2008 Apr 27.

Schroeder P, Krutmann J. What is needed for a sunscreen to provide complete protection. *Skin Therapy Lett*. 2010. 15(4):4-5. Available at: www.skintherapyletter.com/2010/15.4/2.html. Accessed March 19, 2011.

Piazena H, Kelleher DK. Effects of infrared-A irradiation on skin: discrepancies in published data highlight the need for an exact consideration of physical and photobiological laws and appropriate experimental settings. *Photochem Photobiol*. 2010. 86(3):687-705. Epub 2010 Apr 16.

Cho S, Shin MH, Kim YK, et al. Effects of infrared radiation and heat on human skin aging in vivo. *J Investig Dermatol Symp Proc*. 2009. 14(1):15-19. doi:10.1038/jidsymp.2009.7.

301. Piazena H, Kelleher DK. Effects of infrared-A irradiation on skin: discrepancies in published data highlight the need for an exact consideration of physical and photobiological laws and appropriate experimental settings. *Photochem Photobiol*. 2010. 86(3):687-705. Epub 2010 Apr 16.

302. Schroeder P, Calles C, Benesova T, Macaluso F, Krutmann J. Photoprotection beyond ultraviolet radiation–effective sun protection has to include protection against infrared A radiation-induced skin damage. *Skin Pharmacol Physiol*. 2010. 23(1):15-17. Epub 2010 Jan 14.

Piazena H, Kelleher DK. Effects of infrared-A irradiation on skin: discrepancies in published data highlight the need for an exact consideration of physical and photobiological laws and appropriate experimental settings. *Photochem Photobiol*. 2010. 86(3):687-705. Epub 2010 Apr 16.

303. Schroeder P, Haendeler J, Krutmann J. The role of near infrared radiation in photoaging of the skin. *Exp Gerontol*. 2008. 43(7):629-632. Epub 2008 Apr 27.

Schroeder P, Lademann J, Darvin ME, et al. Infrared radiation-induced matrix metalloproteinase in human skin: implications for protection. *J Invest Dermatol*. 2008. 128(10): 2491–2497. Epub 2008 May 1.

304. Schroeder P, Calles C, Benesova T, Macaluso F, Krutmann J. Photoprotection beyond ultraviolet radiation–effective sun protection has to include protection against infrared A radiation-induced skin damage. *Skin Pharmacol Physiol*. 2010. 23(1):15-17. Epub 2010 Jan 14.

Schroeder P, Pohl C, Calles C, Marks C, Wild S, Krutmann J: Cellular response to infrared radiation involves retrograde mitochondrial signaling. *Free Radic Biol Med*. 2007. 43(1):128–135. Epub 2007 Apr 10.

Kang JH. Protective effects of carnosine and homocarnosine on ferritin and hydrogen peroxide-mediated DNA damage. *BMB Rep*. 2010. 43(10):683-687.

305. University of California Riverside Website. Biochemistry and Physiology of Vitamin D. Available at: http://vitamind.ucr.edu/chem.html. Accessed February 2, 2011.

306. Quest Diagnostics Website. Vitamin D, 25-Hydroxy, LC/MS/MS. Available at: www.questdiagnostics.com/hcp/testmenu/jsp/showTestMenu.jsp?fn=17306. html&labCode=AMD. Accessed May 3, 2011.

307. Heaney RP, Recker RR, Grote J, Horst RL, Armas LA. Vitamin D(3) is more potent than vitamin D(2) in humans. *J Clin Endocrinol Metab.* 2011. 96(3):E447-452. Epub 2010 Dec 22.

308. The Telegraph Website. Alleyne R. Vitamin D Health Warning for the Children Who Shun the Sun. Available at: www.telegraph.co.uk/health/healthnews/7995128/Vitamin-D-health-warning-for-the-children-who-shun-the-sun.html#disqus_thread. Accessed February 2, 2011.

309. The Telegraph Website. Smith R. Middle Class Children Suffering Rickets. Available at: www.telegraph.co.uk/health/healthnews/8128781/Middle-class-children-suffering-rickets.html. Accessed February 2, 2011.

310. The Free Medical Dictionary Website. Osteomalacia. Available at: www.medical-dictionary.thefreedictionary.com/osteomalacia. Accessed February 2, 2011.
Dictionary.com Website. Rickets. Available at: http://dictionary.reference.com/browse/rickets. Accessed February 2, 2011.

311. Medscape Today Website. Rickets Reemerging In United States. Available at: www.medscape.com/viewarticle/412104. Accessed February 2, 2011.

312. Hirani V, Tull K, Ali A, Mindell J. Urgent action needed to improve vitamin D status among older people in England! *Age Ageing.* 2010. 39(1):62-68. Epub 2009 Nov 23.

313. Holick MF, Chen TC. Vitamin D deficiency: a worldwide problem with health consequences. *Am J Clin Nutr.* 2008. 87(4):1080S-1086S.

314. Prentice A. Vitamin D deficiency: a global perspective. *Nutr Rev.* 2008. 66(10 Suppl 2):S153-164.

315. Lanham-New SA, Buttriss JL, Miles LM, et al. Proceedings of the Rank Forum on Vitamin D. *Br J Nutr.* 2011. 105(1):144-156. Epub 2010 Dec 7.

316. Grant WB, Mohr SB. Ecological studies of ultraviolet B, vitamin D and cancer since 2000. *Ann Epidemiol.* 2009. 19(7):446-454. Epub 2009 Mar 9.

317. Garland CF, Gorham ED, Grant WB, Garland FC. Ultraviolet B irradiance and vitamin D status are inversely associated with incidence rates of pancreatic cancer worldwide. *Pancreas.* 2010. 39(5):669-674.
Bodiwala D, Luscombe CJ, French ME, et al. Susceptibility to prostate cancer: studies on interactions between UVR exposure and skin type. *Carcinogenesis.* 2003. 24(4):711-717.
Garland CF, Mohr SB, Gorham ED, Grant WB, Garland FC. Role of ultraviolet B irradiance and vitamin D in prevention of ovarian cancer. *Am J Prev Med.* 2006. 31(6):512-514.
Mohr SB, Garland CF, Gorham ED, Grant WB, Garland FC. Is ultraviolet B irradiance inversely associated with incidence rates of endometrial cancer: an ecological study of 107 countries. *Prev Med.* 2007. 45(5):327-331. Epub 2007 Feb 4.
Mohr SB, Garland CF, Gorham ED, Grant WB, Garland FC. Relationship between low ultraviolet B irradiance and higher breast cancer risk in 107 countries. *Breast J.* 2008. 14(3):255-260. Epub 2008 Apr 17.

Mohr SB, Garland CF, Gorham ED, Grant WB, Garland FC. Ultraviolet B
irradiance and incidence rates of bladder cancer in 174 countries. *Am J Prev
Med*. 2010. 38(3):296-302.

Ng K, Wolpin BM, Meyerhardt JA, et al. Prospective study of predictors
of vitamin D status and survival in patients with colorectal cancer. *Br J
Cancer*. 2009. 101(6):916-923. Epub 2009 Aug 18.

Feskanich D, Ma J, Fuchs CS, et al. Plasma vitamin D metabolites and risk of
colorectal cancer in women. *Cancer Epidemiol Biomarkers Prev*. 2004.
13(9):1502-1508.

Garland CF, Gorham ED, Mohr SB, Garland FC. Vitamin D for cancer prevention:
global perspective. *Ann Epidemiol*. 2009. 19(7):468-483.

Giovannucci E, Liu Y, Rimm EB, et al. Prospective study of predictors of
vitamin D status and cancer incidence and mortality in men. *J Natl Cancer
Inst*. 2006. 98(7):451-459.

Grant WB. An estimate of premature cancer mortality in the U.S. due to inadequate
doses of solar ultraviolet-B radiation. *Cancer*. 2002. 94(6):1867-75.

Grant WB. An ecological study of cancer incidence and mortality rates in
France with respect to latitude, an index for vitamin D production.
Dermatoendocrinol. 2010. 2(2):62-67.

Mohr SB, Gorham ED, Garland CF, Grant WB, Garland FC. Low ultraviolet B
and increased risk of brain cancer: an ecological study of 175 countries.
Neuroepidemiology. 2010. 35(4):281-290. Epub 2010 Oct 14.

318. Gamulin M, Znaor A, Fucic A. Increase of hormone-dependent cancer incidence
in population under the age of forty. 2008 ASCO Annual Meeting
Proceedings (Post-Meeting Edition). *J Clin Oncol*. 2008. 26(15S):1518.

319. Garland FC, White MR, Garland CF, Shaw E, Gorham ED. Occupational
sunlight exposure and melanoma in the U.S. Navy. *Arch Environ Health*.
1990. 45(5):261-267.

320. University of California Riverside Website. Biochemistry and Physiology of
Vitamin D. Available at: http://vitamind.ucr.edu/chem.html. Accessed
February 2, 2011.

321. Glossmann HH. Origin of 7-dehydrocholesterol (provitamin D) in the Skin. *J
Invest Dermatol*. 2010. 130(8):2139-2141. Epub 2010 May 6.

Bogh MK, Schmedes AV, Philipsen PA, Thieden E, Wulf HC. Vitamin D
production after UVB exposure depends on baseline vitamin D and
total cholesterol but not on skin pigmentation. *J Invest Dermatol*. 2010.
130(2):546–553. Epub 2009 Oct 8. Erratum in: J Invest Dermatol. 2010.
130(6):1751; Comment in: *J Invest Dermatol*. 2010. 130(2):330; *J Invest
Dermatol*. 2010. 130(2):346–348; *J Invest Dermatol*. 2010. 130(12):2848-
2850; *J Invest Dermatol*. 2010. 130(8):2139-2141.

322. Goldstein MR, Mascitelli L, Pezzetta F. Statin therapy, muscle function and
vitamin D. *QJM*. 2009. 102(12):890-891. Epub 2009 Sep 7.

323. Eyles D, Brown J, Mackay-Sim A, McGrath J, Feron F. Vitamin D3 and brain
development. *Neuroscience*. 2003. 118(3):641-653.

Holick MF. Vitamin D Deficiency. *N Engl J Med*. 2007. 357(3):266-281.
Comment in: *N Engl J Med*. 2007. 357(19):1980-1981. Author reply 1981-
1982; *N Engl J Med*. 2007. 357(19):1981. Author reply 1981-1982; *Int J
Clin Pract*. 2009. 63(8):1265; N Engl J Med. 2007. 357(19):1981. Author
reply 1981-1982; *N Engl J Med*. 2007. 357(19):1981. Author reply 1981-
1982.

Holick MF. Resurrection of vitamin D deficiency and rickets. *J Clin Invest*. 2006. 116(8):2062-2072.

Holick MF, Garabedian M. Vitamin D: photobiology, metabolism, mechanism of action, and clinical applications. In: *Primer on the Metabolic Bone Diseases and Disorders of Mineral Metabolism*. 6th ed. Washington, DC: American Society for Bone and Mineral Research. 2006. Pages 129-137. Cited in Holick MF. Vitamin D Deficiency. *N Engl J Med*. 2007. 357(3):266-281.

Bouillon R. Vitamin D: from photosynthesis, metabolism, and action to clinical applications. In: DeGroot LJ, Jameson JL, eds. *Endocrinology*. W.B. Saunders, Philadelphia. 2001. Pages 1009-1028.

DeLuca HF. Overview of general physiologic features and functions of vitamin D. *Am J Clin Nutr*. 2004. 80:Suppl:1689S-1696S. Cited in Holick MF. Vitamin D Deficiency. N Engl J Med. 2007. 357(3):266-281.

Dusso AS, Brown AJ, Slatopolsky E. Vitamin D. *Am J Physiol Renal Physiol*. 2005;289:F8-F28. Cited in Holick MF. Vitamin D Deficiency. *N Engl J Med*. 2007. 357(3):266-281.

MacDonald P. Molecular biology of the vitamin D receptor. In: Holick MF, ed. Vitamin D: Physiology, Molecular Biology, and Clinical Applications. Totowa, NJ: Humana Press. 1999. Pages109–128.

324. Holick MF. Resurrection of vitamin D deficiency and rickets. *J Clin Invest*. 2006. 116(8):2062-2072.

325. Bouillon R. Vitamin D: from photosynthesis, metabolism, and action to clinical applications. In: DeGroot LJ, Jameson JL, eds. *Endocrinology*. W.B. Saunders, Philadelphia. 2001. Pages 1009-1028. Cited in Holick MF. Vitamin D Deficiency. *N Engl J Med*. 2007. 357(3):266-281. Comment in: *N Engl J Med*. 2007. 357(19):1980-1981. Author reply 1981-1982; *N Engl J Med*. 2007. 357(19):1981. Author reply 1981-1982; *Int J Clin Pract*. 2009. 63(8):1265; *N Engl J Med*. 2007. 357(19):1981. Author reply 1981-1982; *N Engl J Med*. 2007. 357(19):1981. Author reply 1981-1982.

326. Holick MF, Chen TC. Vitamin D deficiency: a worldwide problem with health consequences. *Am J Clin Nutr*. 2008. 87(4):1080S-1086S.

327. Trémezaygues L, Reichrath J. From the bench to emerging new clinical concepts: Our present understanding of the importance of the vitamin D endocrine system (VDES) for skin cancer. *Dermatoendocrinol*. 2011. 3(1):11-17.

Chakraborti CK. Vitamin D as a promising anticancer agent. *Indian J Pharmacol*. 2011. 43(2):113-120.

Zheng Y, Zhou H, Ooi LL, Snir AD, Dunstan CR, Seibel MJ. Vitamin D deficiency promotes prostate cancer growth in bone. *Prostate*. 2011. 71(9):1012-1021. doi: 10.1002/pros.21316. Epub 2010 Dec 28.

Gueli N, Verrusio W, Linguanti A, et al. Vitamin D: drug of the future. A new therapeutic approach. *Arch Gerontol Geriatr*. 2011 Mar 31. [Epub ahead of print].

328. Kivity S, Agmon-Levin N, Zisappl M, et al. Vitamin D and autoimmune thyroid diseases. *Cell Mol Immunol*. 2011. 8(3):243-247. Epub 2011 Jan 31.

329. Burgaz A, Orsini N, Larsson SC, Wolk A. Blood 25-hydroxyvitamin D concentration and hypertension: a meta-analysis. *J Hypertens*. 2011. 29(4)636-645. Epub ahead of print.

330. Zittermann A. Vitamin D and disease prevention with special reference to cardiovascular disease. *Prog Biophys Mol Biol*. 2006. 92(1):39-48. Epub 2006 Feb 28.

331. Pilz S, Tomaschitz A, Drechsler C, Zittermann A, Dekker JM, März W. Vitamin D supplementation: a promising approach for the prevention and treatment of strokes. *Curr Drug Targets*. 2011. 12(1):88-96.

332. Schwalfenberg GK. A review of the critical role of vitamin D in the functioning of the immune system and the clinical implications of vitamin D deficiency. *Mol Nutr Food Res*. 2011. 55(1):96-108. doi: 10.1002/mnfr.201000174. Epub 2010 Sep 7.

Bartley J. Vitamin D, innate immunity and upper respiratory tract infection. *J Laryngol Otol*. 2010. 124(5):465-469. Epub 2010 Jan 13.

Ginde AA, Mansbach JM, Camargo CA Jr. Vitamin D, respiratory infections, and asthma. *Curr Allergy Asthma Rep*. 2009. 9(1):81-87.

333. Medscape Today Website. Barclay L. Vitamin D Deficiency Linked to Bacterial Vaginosis. Available at: www.medscape.com/viewarticle/703577. Accessed February 2, 2011.

334. Wang Y, Deluca HF. Is the vitamin d receptor found in muscle? *Endocrinology*. 2011. 152(2):354-363. Epub 2010 Dec 29.

Schubert L, DeLuca HF. Hypophosphatemia is responsible for skeletal muscle weakness of vitamin D deficiency. *Arch Biochem Biophys*. 2010. 500(2):157-161. Epub 2010 May 31.

Halliday TM, Peterson NJ, Thomas JJ, Kleppinger K, Hollis BW, Larson-Meyer DE. Vitamin D status relative to diet, lifestyle, injury, and illness in college athletes. *Med Sci Sports Exerc*. 2011. 43(2):335-343.

335. Medscape Today Website. Barclay L. Higher Vitamin D Levels Linked to Lower Risk for Female Pelvic Floor Disorders? Available at: www.medscape.com/viewarticle/719592. Accessed February 2, 2011.

336. Dixon KM, Mason RS. Vitamin D. *Int J Biochem Cell Biol*. 2009. 41(5):982-985. Epub 2008 Aug 3.

Plotnikoff GA, Quigley JM. Prevalence of severe hypovitaminosis D in patients with persistent, nonspecific musculoskeletal pain. *Mayo Clin Proc*. 2003. 78(12):1463-1470. Comments in: *Mayo Clin Proc*. 2004. 79(12):1585-6; author reply 1586-1587; *Mayo Clin Proc*. 2003. 78(12):1457-1459; *Mayo Clin Proc*. 2004. 79(5):696, 699; author reply 699; *Mayo Clin Proc*. 2004. 79(5):695; author reply 695-696; *Mayo Clin Proc*. 2004. 79(5):694; author reply 694-695.

337. Medscape Today Website. Barclay L. Vitamin D Deficiency Linked to Greater Risk for Primary Cesarean Delivery. Available at: www.medscape.com/viewarticle/585864. Accessed February 2, 2011.

338. Ganji V, Milone C, Cody MM, McCarty F, Wang YT. Serum vitamin D concentrations are related to depression in young adult US population: the Third National Health and Nutrition Examination Survey. *Int Arch Med*. 2010. 3:29.

339. Gloth FM III, Alam W, Hollis B. Vitamin D vs. broad spectrum phototherapy in the treatment of seasonal effective disorder. *J Nutr Health Aging*. 1999. 3(1):5-7.

340. Kayaniyil S, Vieth R, Harris SB, et al. Association of 25(OH)D and PTH with metabolic syndrome and its traditional and nontraditional components. *J Clin Endocrinol Metab*. 2011. 96(1):168-175. Epub 2010 Oct 27.

341. Lagunova Z, Porojnicu AC, Vieth R, Lindberg FA, Hexeberg S, Moan J. Serum 25-hydroxyvitamin D is a predictor of serum 1,25-dihydroxyvitamin D in overweight and obese patients. *J Nutr*. 2011. 141(1):112-117. Epub 2010 Nov 17.

Macdonald HM, Mavroeidi A, Barr RJ, Black AJ, Fraser WD, Reid DM. Vitamin D status in postmenopausal women living at higher latitudes in the UK in relation to bone health, overweight, sunlight exposure and dietary vitamin D. *Bone.* 2008. 42(5):996-1003. Epub 2008 Feb 9.

342. Lindqvist PG, Olsson H, Landin-Olsson M. Are active sun exposure habits related to lowering risk of type 2 diabetes mellitus in women, a prospective cohort study? *Diabetes Res Clin Pract.* 2010. 90(1):109-114.

Penckofer S, Kouba J, Wallis DE, Emanuele MA. Vitamin D and diabetes: let the sunshine in. *Diabetes Educ.* 2008. 34(6):939-940, 942, 944 passim.

Kayaniyil S, Vieth R, Retnakaran R, et al. Association of vitamin D with insulin resistance and beta-cell dysfunction in subjects at risk for type 2 diabetes. *Diabetes Care.* 2010. 33(6):1379-1381. Epub 2010 Mar 9.

343. Levin AD, Wadhera V, Leach ST, et al. Vitamin D deficiency in children with inflammatory bowel disease. *Dig Dis Sci.* 2011. 56 Jan (3):830-836. Epub 2011 Jan 11.

344. Jørgensen SP, Agnholt J, Glerup H, et al. Clinical trial: vitamin D3 treatment in Crohn's disease - a randomized double-blind placebo-controlled study. *Aliment Pharmacol Ther.* 2010. 32(3):377-383. Epub 2010 May 11.

345. Ryan C, Moran B, McKenna MJ, et al. The effect of narrowband UVB treatment for psoriasis on vitamin D status during wintertime in Ireland. *Arch Dermatol.* 2010. 146(8):836-842. Erratum in: *Arch Dermatol.* 2010. 146(11):1282.

Kurian A, Barankin B. Current effective topical therapies in the management of psoriasis. *Skin Therapy Lett.* 2011. 16(1):4-7.

346. Annweiler C, Schott AM, Rolland Y, Blain H, Herrmann FR, Beauchet O. Dietary intake of vitamin D and cognition in older women: a large population-based study. *Neurology.* 2010. 75(20):1810-1816.

347. Salzer J, Svenningsson A, Sundström P. Season of birth and multiple sclerosis in Sweden. *Acta Neurol Scand.* 2010. 122(1):70-73. Corrected and republished: Acta Neurol Scand. 2010. 121(1):20-23.

348. McGrath J, Brown A, St Clair D. Prevention and schizophrenia--the role of dietary factors. *Schizophr Bull.* 2011. 37(2):272-283. Epub 2010 Oct 25.

McGrath JJ, Eyles DW, Pedersen CB, et al. Neonatal vitamin D status and risk of schizophrenia: a population-based case-control study. *Arch Gen Psychiatry.* 2010. 67(9):889-894.

McGrath J, Selten JP, Chant D. Long-term trends in sunshine duration and its association with schizophrenia birth rates and age at first registration–data from Australia and the Netherlands. *Schizophr Res.* 2002. 54(3):199-212.

349. Mohr SB, Garland CF, Gorham ED, Garland FC. The association between ultraviolet B irradiance, vitamin D status and incidence rates of type 1 diabetes in 51 regions worldwide. *Diabetologia.* 2008. 51(8):1391-1398. Epub 2008 Jun 12.

Hyppönen E. Vitamin D and increasing incidence of type 1 diabetes-evidence for an association? *Diabetes Obes Metab.* 2010. 12(9):737-743.

Hypponen E, Laara E, Reunanen A, Jarvelin M-R, Virtanen SM. Intake of vitamin D and risk of type 1 diabetes: a birth-cohort study. *Lancet.* 2001. 358(9292):1500-1503.

350. Holick MF. Vitamin D Deficiency. *N Engl J Med*. 2007. 357(3):266-281. Comment in: *N Engl J Med*. 2007. 357(19):1980-1981. Author reply 1981-1982; *N Engl J Med*. 2007. 357(19):1981. Author reply 1981-1982; *Int J Clin Pract*. 2009. 63(8):1265; *N Engl J Med*. 2007. 357(19):1981. Author reply 1981-1982; *N Engl J Med*. 2007. 357(19):1981. Author reply 1981-1982.

Holick MF, Garabedian M. Vitamin D: photobiology, metabolism, mechanism of action, and clinical applications. In: *Primer on the metabolic bone diseases and disorders of mineral metabolism*. 6th ed. Washington, DC: American Society for Bone and Mineral Research. 2006. Pages 129-137.

Bouillon R. Vitamin D: from photosynthesis, metabolism, and action to clinical applications. In: DeGroot LJ, Jameson JL, eds. *Endocrinology*. W.B. Saunders, Philadelphia. 2001. Pages 1009-1028. Cited in Holick MF. Vitamin D Deficiency. *N Engl J Med*. 2007. 357(3):266-281.

DeLuca HF. Overview of general physiologic features and functions of vitamin D. *Am J Clin Nutr*. 2004. 80(6 Suppl):1689S-1696S. Cited in Holick MF. Vitamin D Deficiency. *N Engl J Med*. 2007. 357(3):266-281. Comment in: *N Engl J Med*. 2007. 357(19):1980-1981. Author reply 1981-1982; *N Engl J Med*. 2007. 357(19):1981. Author reply 1981-1982; *Int J Clin Pract*. 2009. 63(8):1265; *N Engl J Med*. 2007. 357(19):1981. Author reply 1981-1982; *N Engl J Med*. 2007. 357(19):1981. Author reply 1981-1982. Cited in Holick MF. Vitamin D Deficiency. *N Engl J Med*. 2007. 357(3):266-281.

351. wordiQ Website. Vitamin D – Definition. Available at: www.wordiq.com/definition/Vitamin_D. Accessed February 2, 2011.

Hollis BW. Circulating 25-hydroxyvitamin D levels indicative of vitamin D sufficiency: implications for establishing a new effective dietary intake recommendation for vitamin D. *J Nutr*. 2005. 135(2):317-322.

Oregon State University Website. Higdon J. Calcium. Available at: http://lpi.oregonstate.edu/infocenter/minerals/calcium/index.html/. Accessed June 19, 2011.

352. Cavalier E, Rozet E, Gadisseur R, et al. Measurement uncertainty of 25-OH vitamin D determination with different commercially available kits: impact on the clinical cut offs. *Osteoporos Int*. 2010. 21(6):1047-51. Epub 2009 Sep 9.

353. Vogeser M. Quantification of circulating 25-hydroxyvitamin D by liquid chromatography-tandem mass spectrometry. *J Steroid Biochem Mol Biol*. 2010. 121(3-5):565-73. Epub 2010 Mar 4.

354. Holick MF. Vitamin D: a d-lightful health perspective. *Nutr Rev*. 2008. 66(10 Suppl 2):S182-194.

Burgaz A, Akesson A, Michaëlsson K, Wolk A. 25-hydroxyvitamin D accumulation during summer in elderly women at latitude 60 degrees N. *J Intern Med*. 2009. 266(5):476-483. Epub 2009 Apr 27.

355. Holick MF. Vitamin D Deficiency. *N Engl J Med*. 2007. 357(3):266-281. Comment in: *N Engl J Med*. 2007. 357(19):1980-1981. Author reply 1981-1982; *N Engl J Med*. 2007. 357(19):1981. Author reply 1981-1982; *Int J Clin Pract*. 2009. 63(8):1265; *N Engl J Med*. 2007. 357(19):1981. Author reply 1981-1982; *N Engl J Med*. 2007. 357(19):1981. Author reply 1981-1982.

Holick MF. High prevalence of vitamin D inadequacy and implications for health. *Mayo Clin Proc*. 2006. 81(3):353-373. Cited in Holick MF. Vitamin D Deficiency. *N Engl J Med*. 2007. 357(3):266-281.

Bischoff-Ferrari HA, Giovannucci E, Willett WC, Dietrich T, Dawson-Hughes B. Estimation of optimal serum concentrations of 25-hydroxyvitamin D for multiple health outcomes. *Am J Clin Nutr*. 2006. 84(1):18-28. Erratum, *Am J Clin Nutr*. 2006. 84(5):1253 and Am J Clin Nutr. 2007. 86(3):809. Cited in Holick MF. Vitamin D Deficiency. *N Engl J Med*. 2007. 357(3):266-281.

Malabanan A, Veronikis IE, Holick MF. Redefining vitamin D insufficiency. *Lancet*. 1998. 351(9105):805-806. Cited in Holick MF. Vitamin D Deficiency. *N Engl J Med*. 2007. 357(3):266-281.

Thomas MK, Lloyd-Jones DM, Thadhani RI, et al. Hypovitaminosis D in medical inpatients. *N Engl J Med*. 1998. 338(12):777-783. Cited in Holick MF. Vitamin D Deficiency. *N Engl J Med*. 2007. 357(3):266-281.

Charzewska J, Chlebna-Sokół D, Chybicka A, et al. Recommendations of prophylaxis of vitamin D deficiency in Poland (2009). *Med Wieku Rozwoj*. 2010. 14(2):218-223.

Bischoff-Ferrari HA, Shao A, Dawson-Hughes B, Hathcock J, Giovannucci E, Willett WC. Benefit-risk assessment of vitamin D supplementation. *Osteoporos Int*. 2010. 21(7):1121-1132. Epub 2009 Dec 3.

Dawson-Hughes B, Heaney RP, Holick MF, Lips P, Meunier PJ, Vieth R. Estimates of optimal vitamin D status. *Osteoporos Int*. 2005. 16(7):713-716. Epub 2005 Mar 18.

356. Ashwell M, Stone EM, Stolte H, et al. UK Food Standards Agency Workshop Report: an investigation of the relative contributions of diet and sunlight to vitamin D status. *Br J Nutr*. 2010. 104(4):603-611. Epub 2010 Jun 4.

357. MacLaughlin J, Holick MF. Aging decreases the capacity of human skin to produce vitamin D3. *J Clin Invest*. 1985. 76(4):1536-1538.

Holick MF. Environmental factors that influence the cutaneous production of vitamin D. *Am J Clin Nutr*. 1995. 61(3 suppl):638S-645S.

Holick MF, Matsuoka LY, Wortsman J. Age, vitamin D, and solar ultraviolet. *Lancet*. 1989. 2(8671):1104–1105.

358. Chen TC, Chimeh F, Lu Z, et. al. Factors that influence the cutaneous synthesis and dietary sources of vitamin D. *Arch Biohem Biophys*. 2007. 460(2):213-217.

Brenner M, Hearing VJ. The protective role of melanin against UV damage in human skin. *Photochem Photobiol*. 2008. 84(3):539-549.

Tian XQ, Chen TC, Matsuoka LY, Wortsman J, Holick MF. Kinetic and thermodynamic studies of the conversion of previtamin D3 to vitamin D3 in human skin. *J Biol Chem*. 1993. 268(20):14888-14892.

359. Hall LM, Kimlin MG, Aronov PA, et al. Vitamin D intake needed to maintain target serum 25-hydroxyvitamin D concentrations in participants with low sun exposure and dark skin pigmentation is substantially higher than current recommendations. *J Nutr*. 2010. 140(3):542-550. Epub 2010 Jan 6.

Talwar SA, Aloia JF, Pollack S, Yeh JK. Dose response to vitamin D supplementation among postmenopausal African American women. *Am J Clin Nutr*. 2007. 86(6):1657-1662.

360. Mayo Clinic Website. Vitamin D. Available at: www.mayoclinic.com/health/vitamin-d/NS_patient-vitamind. Accessed February 2, 2011.

361. Holick MF. Photosynthesis of vitamin D in the skin: effect of environmental and life-style variables. *Fed Proc*. 1987. 46(5):1876-1882.

Webb AR, DeCosta BR, Holick MF. Sunlight regulates the production of vitamin D by causing its photodegradation. *J Clin Endocrinol Metabol*. 1989. 68:882–887.

362. Ashwell M, Stone EM, Stolte H, et al. UK Food Standards Agency Workshop Report: an investigation of the relative contributions of diet and sunlight to vitamin D status. *Br J Nutr*. 2010. 104(4):603-611. Epub 2010 Jun 4.

363. Terushkin V, Bender A, Psaty EL, Engelsen O, Wang SQ, Halpern AC. Estimated equivalency of vitamin D production from natural sun exposure versus oral vitamin D supplementation across seasons at two US latitudes. *J Am Acad Dermatol*. 2010. 62(6):929.e1-9. Epub 2010 Apr 3.

364. Holick MF. Environmental factors that influence the cutaneous production of vitamin D. *Am J Clin Nutr*. 1995. 61(3 suppl):638S-645S.

365. Mayo Clinic Website. Vitamin D. Available at: www.mayoclinic.com/health/vitamin-d/NS_patient-vitamind. Accessed February 2, 2011.

366. Rhodes LE, Webb AR, Fraser HI, et al. Recommended summer sunlight exposure levels can produce sufficient (> or =20 ng ml(-1)) but not the proposed optimal (> or =32 ng ml(-1)) 25(OH)D levels at UK latitudes. *J Invest Dermatol*. 2010. 130(5):1411-1418. Epub 2010 Jan 14.

367. Ashwell M, Stone EM, Stolte H, et al. UK Food Standards Agency Workshop Report: an investigation of the relative contributions of diet and sunlight to vitamin D status. *Br J Nutr*. 2010. 104(4):603-611. Epub 2010 Jun 4.

368. Burgaz A, Akesson A, Michaëlsson K, Wolk A. 25-hydroxyvitamin D accumulation during summer in elderly women at latitude 60 degrees N. J Intern Med. 2009. 266(5):476-483. Epub 2009 Apr 27.

369. Webb AR, Kift R, Durkin MT, et al. The role of sunlight exposure in determining the vitamin D status of the U.K. white adult population. *Br J Dermatol*. 2010. 163(5):1050-1055. doi: 10.1111/j.1365-2133.2010.09975.x. Epub 2010 Sep 30.

370. Ashwell M, Stone EM, Stolte H, et al. UK Food Standards Agency Workshop Report: an investigation of the relative contributions of diet and sunlight to vitamin D status. *Br J Nutr*. 2010. 104(4):603-611. Epub 2010 Jun 4.

371. Diffey BL. Is casual exposure to summer sunlight effective at maintaining adequate vitamin D status? *Photodermatol Photoimmunol Photomed*. 2010. 26(4):172–176.

372. Diffey BL. Sunscreens as a preventative measure in melanoma: an evidence-based approach or the precautionary principle? *Br J Dermatol*. 2009. 161(Suppl. 3):25–27.

373. Webb AR, Engelsen O. Calculated ultraviolet exposure levels for a healthy vitamin D status. *Photochem Photobiol*. 2006. 82(6):1697–1703.
    Ashwell M, Stone EM, Stolte H, et al. UK Food Standards Agency Workshop Report: an investigation of the relative contributions of diet and sunlight to vitamin D status. *Br J Nutr*. 2010. 104(4):603-611. Epub 2010 Jun 4.

374. Mayo Clinic Website. Vitamin D and Related Compounds (Oral Route, Parenteral Route). Available at: http://www.mayoclinic.com/health/drug-information/DR602171/METHOD=print&DSECTION=all. Accessed June 19, 2011.

375. Holick MF, Chen TC. Vitamin D deficiency: a worldwide problem with health consequences. *Am J Clin Nutr*. 2008. 87(4):1080S-1086S.

376. University of California Riverside Website. Nutritional Aspects of Vitamin D. Available at: http://vitamind.ucr.edu/nutri.html. Accessed June 13, 2011
    Holick MF. Vitamin D Deficiency. *N Engl J Med*. 2007. 357(3):266-281.
    Holick MF, Chen TC. Vitamin D deficiency: a worldwide problem with health consequences. *Am J Clin Nutr*. 2008. 87(4):1080S-1086S.
    wordiQ Website. Vitamin D – Definition. Available at: www.wordiq.com/definition/Vitamin_D. Accessed June 12, 2011.

377. University of California Riverside Website. Nutritional Aspects of Vitamin D. Available at: http://vitamind.ucr.edu/nutri.html. Accessed June 13, 2011

378. Colorado State University Website. Bowan R. Vitamin D (Calcitriol). Available at: www.vivo.colostate.edu/hbooks/pathphys/endocrine/otherendo/vitamind. html. Accessed June 13, 2011.

379. Ross AC, Manson JE, Abrams SA, et al. The 2011 report on dietary reference intakes for calcium and vitamin D from the Institute of Medicine: what clinicians need to know. *J Clin Endocrinol Metab*. 2011. 96(1):53-58. Epub 2010 Nov 29. Comment in: *J Clin Endocrinol Metab*. 2011. 96(1):69-71.

380. Heaney RP, Holick MF. Why the IOM recommendations for vitamin D are deficient. *J Bone Miner Res*. 2011. 26(3):455-457.

381. Heaney RP, Davies KM, Chen TC, Holick MF, Barger-Lux MJ. Human serum 25-hydroxycholecalciferol response to extended oral dosing with cholecalciferol. *Am J Clin Nutr*. 2003. 77(1):204-210.

382. Holick MF. Vitamin D Deficiency. *N Engl J Med*. 2007. 357(3):266-281. Comment in: *N Engl J Med*. 2007. 357(19):1980-1981. Author reply 1981-1982; *N Engl J Med*. 2007. 357(19):1981. Author reply 1981-1982; *Int J Clin Pract*. 2009. 63(8):1265; *N Engl J Med*. 2007. 357(19):1981. Author reply 1981-1982; *N Engl J Med*. 2007. 357(19):1981. Author reply 1981-1982.

Hollis BW, Wagner CL. Assessment of dietary vitamin D requirements during pregnancy and lactation. *Am J Clin Nutr*. 2004. 79(5):717-726. Cited in Holick MF. Vitamin D Deficiency. *N Engl J Med*. 2007. 357(3):266-281.

Lee JM, Smith JR, Philipp BL, Chen TC, Mathieu J, Holick MF. Vitamin D deficiency in a healthy group of mothers and newborn infants. Clin Pediatr (Phila). 2007. 46(1):42-44. Cited in Holick MF. Vitamin D Deficiency. *N Engl J Med*. 2007. 357(3):266-281.

Bodnar LM, Simhan HN, Powers RW, Frank MP, Cooperstein E, Roberts JM. High prevalence of vitamin D insufficiency in black and white pregnant women residing in the northern United States and their neonates. *J Nutr*. 2007. 137(2):447-452. Cited in Holick MF. Vitamin D Deficiency. N Engl J Med. 2007. 357(3):266-281.

383. Macdonald HM, Mavroeidi A, Barr RJ, Black AJ, Fraser WD, Reid DM. Vitamin D status in postmenopausal women living at higher latitudes in the UK in relation to bone health, overweight, sunlight exposure and dietary vitamin D. *Bone*. 2008. 42(5):996-1003. Epub 2008 Feb 9.

Charzewska J, Chlebna-Sokół D, Chybicka A, et al. Recommendations of prophylaxis of vitamin D deficiency in Poland (2009). *Med Wieku Rozwoj*. 2010. 14(2):218-223.

Cashman KD, Hill TR, Lucey AJ, et al. Estimation of the dietary requirement for vitamin D in healthy adults. *Am J Clin Nutr*. 2008. 88(6):1535-1542.

Holick MF, Chen TC. Vitamin D deficiency: a worldwide problem with health consequences. *Am J Clin Nutr*. 2008. 87(4):1080S-1086S.

Holick MF. Vitamin D: a d-lightful health perspective. *Nutr Rev*. 2008. 66(10 Suppl 2):S182-194.

Bischoff-Ferrari HA, Giovannucci E, Willett WC, Dietrich T, Dawson-Hughes B. Estimation of optimal serum concentrations of 25-hydroxyvitamin D for multiple health outcomes. *Am J Clin Nutr*. 2006. 84(1):18-28. Erratum, *Am J Clin Nutr*. 2006. 84(5):1253 and *Am J Clin Nutr*. 2007. 86(3):809.

384. Aloia JF, Patel M, Dimaano R, et al. Vitamin D intake to attain a desired serum 25-hydroxyvitamin D concentration. *Am J Clin Nutr.* 2008. 87(6):1952-1958.
385. Moyad MA. Vitamin D: A Rapid Review. *Dermatol Nursing.* 2009. 21(1). Available at: www.medscape.com/viewarticle/589256.
386. Hall LM, Kimlin MG, Aronov PA, et al. Vitamin D intake needed to maintain target serum 25-hydroxyvitamin D concentrations in participants with low sun exposure and dark skin pigmentation is substantially higher than current recommendations. *J Nutr.* 2010. 140(3):542-550. Epub 2010 Jan 6.
387. Talwar SA, Aloia JF, Pollack S, Yeh JK. Dose response to vitamin D supplementation among postmenopausal African American women. *Am J Clin Nutr.* 2007. 86(6):1657-1662.
388. Charzewska J, Chlebna-Sokół D, Chybicka A, et al. Recommendations of prophylaxis of vitamin D deficiency in Poland (2009). *Med Wieku Rozwoj.* 2010. 14(2):218-223.
389. Mayo Clinic Website. Vitamin D: Dosing. Available at: www.mayoclinic.com/health/vitamin-d/NS_patient-vitamind/DSECTION=dosing. Accessed February 2, 2011.
390. Merck Manual Website. Vitamin D. Available at: www.merckmanuals.com/professional/sec01/ch004/ch004k.html. Accessed January 31, 2011.
391. Bogh MK, Schmedes AV, Philipsen PA, Thieden E, Wulf HC. Vitamin D production after UVB exposure depends on baseline vitamin D and total cholesterol but not on skin pigmentation. *J Invest Dermatol.* 2010. 130(2):546–553. Epub 2009 Oct 8. Erratum in: J Invest Dermatol. 2010. 130(6):1751; Comment in: *J Invest Dermatol.* 2010. 130(2):330; *J Invest Dermatol.* 2010. 130(2):346–348; *J Invest Dermatol.* 2010. 130(12):2848-2850; *J Invest Dermatol.* 2010. 130(8):2139-2141.
    Camacho I, Tzu J, Kirsner RS. Regulation of Vitamin D production is independent of skin color. *J Invest Dermatol.* 2010. 130(2):330. doi:10.1038/jid.2009.407. Comment in: *J Invest Dermatol.* 2010. 130(2):546-553.
    Glossmann HH. Origin of 7-dehydrocholesterol (provitamin D) in the Skin. *J Invest Dermatol.* 2010. 130. p (8):2140-2141. Epub 2010 May 6.
392. Norval M, Wulf HC. Does chronic sunscreen use reduce vitamin D production to insufficient levels? *Br J Dermatol.* 2009. 161(4):732-736. Epub 2009 Jun 4. Comment in: *Br J Dermatol.* 2010. 162(3):697. Available at: http://www.medscape.com/viewarticle/713721. Accessed February11, 2011.
    Sayre RM, Dowdy JC. Darkness at noon: sunscreens and vitamin D3. *Photochem Photobiol.* 2007. 83(2):459-463.
    Matsuoka LY, Ide L, Wortsman J, MacLaughlin JA, Holick MF. Sunscreens suppress cutaneous vitamin D3 synthesis. *J Clin Endocrinol Metab.* 1987. 64(6):1165-1168.
393. Bissonnette, R. Update on sunscreens. Skin Therapy Letter. 2008. 13(6):5-7. Available at: www.medscape.com/viewarticle/582990. Accessed June 12, 2011.
394. Holick MF. Vitamin D Deficiency. *N Engl J Med.* 2007. 357(3):266-281. Comment in: *N Engl J Med.* 2007. 357(19):1980-1981. Author reply 1981-1982; *N Engl J Med.* 2007. 357(19):1981. Author reply 1981-1982; Int J Clin Pract. 2009. 63(8):1265; *N Engl J Med.* 2007. 357(19):1981. Author reply 1981-1982; *N Engl J Med.* 2007. 357(19):1981. Author reply 1981-1982.

Holick MF. Resurrection of vitamin D deficiency and rickets. *J Clin Invest*. 2006. 116(8):2062-2072. Cited in Holick MF. Vitamin D Deficiency. *N Engl J Med*. 2007. 357(3):266-281.

Holick MF. Vitamin D: photobiology, metabolism, mechanism of action, and clinical applications. In: Favus M, ed. *Primer on the Metabolic Bone Diseases and Disorders of Mineral Metabolism*. 5th ed. Washington, DC. American Society for Bone and Mineral Research. 2003. Pages 129–137. Cited in Holick MF. Vitamin D Deficiency. *N Engl J Med*. 2007. 357(3):266-281.

Bouillon R. Vitamin D: from photosynthesis, metabolism, and action to clinical applications. In: DeGroot LJ, Jameson JL, eds. *Endocrinology*. W.B. Saunders, Philadelphia. 2001. Pages 1009-1028. Cited in Holick MF. Vitamin D Deficiency. *N Engl J Med*. 2007. 357(3):266-281.

Holick MF. High prevalence of vitamin D inadequacy and implications for health. *Mayo Clin Proc*. 2006. 81(3):353-373. Cited in Holick MF. Vitamin D Deficiency. *N Engl J Med*. 2007. 357(3):266-281.

Holick MF. Vitamin D: importance in the prevention of cancers, type 1 diabetes, heart disease, and osteoporosis. *Am J Clin Nutr*. 2004. 79(3):362-371. Erratum in *Am J Clin Nutr*. 2004. 79(5):890. Cited in Holick MF. Vitamin D Deficiency. *N Engl J Med*. 2007. 357(3):266-281.

395. Grant WB. Solar ultraviolet irradiance and cancer incidence and mortality. *Adv Exp Med Biol*. 2008. 624:16-30.

396. Holick MF. Sunlight, UV-radiation, vitamin D and skin cancer: how much sunlight do we need? *Adv Exp Med Biol*. 2008. 624:1-15.

397. Holick MF. Sunlight, UV-radiation, vitamin D and skin cancer: how much sunlight do we need? *Adv Exp Med Biol*. 2008. 624:1-15.

398. University of California Riverside Website. Biochemistry and Physiology of Vitamin D. Available at: http://vitamind.ucr.edu/nutri.html. Accessed June 12, 2011.

399. Weggemans RM, Schaafsma G, Kromhout D. Towards an adequate intake of vitamin D. An advisory report of the Health Council of the Netherlands. *Eur J Clin Nutr*. 2009. 63(12):1455-1457. Epub 2009 Jul 22. Comment in: *Eur J Clin Nutr*. 2010. 64(6):655; Author reply 656.

400. Shapira N. Nutritional approach to sun protection: a suggested complement to external strategies. Nutr Rev. 68(2):75–86.

401. Nichols JA, Katiyar SK. Skin photoprotection by natural polyphenols: anti-inflammatory, antioxidant and DNA repair mechanisms. *Arch Dermatol Res*. 2010. 302(2):71-83. Epub 2009 Nov 7.

402. Darvin ME, Haag S, Meinke M, Zastrow L, Sterry W, Lademann J. Radical production by infrared A irradiation in human tissue. *Skin Pharmacol Physiol*. 2010. 23(1):40–46. Epub 2010 Jan 14.

403. Fuchs J. Potentials and limitations of the natural antioxidants RRR-alpha-tocopherol, L-ascorbic acid and beta-carotene in cutaneous photoprotection. *Free Radic Biol Med*. 1998. 25(7):848-873.

Greul AK, Grundmann JU, Heinrich F, et al. Photoprotection of UV-irradiated human skin: an antioxidative combination of vitamins E and C, carotenoids, selenium and proanthocyanidins. *Skin Pharmacol Appl Skin Physiol*. 2002. 15(5):307-315.

Shapira N. Nutritional approach to sun protection: a suggested complement to external strategies. *Nutr Rev*. 68(2):75–86.

Boelsma E, Hendriks HF, Roza L. Nutritional skin care: health effects of micronutrients and fatty acids. *Am J Clin Nutr*. 2001. 73(5):853-864.

Dinkova-Kostova AT. Phytochemicals as protectors against ultraviolet radiation: versatility of effects and mechanisms. *Planta Med*. 2008. 74(13):1548–1559. Epub 2008 Aug 11.

404. Biology Online Website. Tedesco AC, Martinez L, Gonzalez S. Photochemistry of UV-induced erythema: Studies on free radical generation and the production of ROS - Photochemistry and photobiology of actinic erythema: defensive and reparative cutaneous mechanisms. Available at: www.biology-online.org/articles/photochemistry_photobiology_actinic_erythema/photochemistry_uv-induced_erythema_studies.html. Accessed June 19, 2011.

405. Darvin ME, Patzelt A, Knorr F, Blume-Peytavi U, Sterry W, Lademann J. One-year study on the variation of carotenoid antioxidant substances in living human skin: influence of dietary supplementation and stress factors. *J Biomed Opt*. 2008. 13(4):044028.

406. Heinrich U, Neukam K, Tronnier H, Sies H, Stahl W. Long-term ingestion of high flavanol cocoa provides photoprotection against UV-induced erythema and improves skin condition in women. *J Nutr*. 2006. 136(6):1565-1569.

407. Darvin ME, Haag SF, Meinke MC, Sterry W, Lademann J. Determination of the influence of IR radiation on the antioxidative network of the human skin. J Biophotonics. 2011. 4(1–2):21–29. doi: 10.1002/jbio.200900111. Epub 2010 Feb 11.

408. Mohasseb M, Ebied S, Yehia MA, Hussein N. Testicular oxidative damage and role of combined antioxidant supplementation in experimental diabetic rats. *J Physiol Biochem*. 2010 Dec 24. [Epub ahead of print].

Ghosh N, Ghosh R, Mandal V, Mandal SC. Recent advances in herbal medicine for treatment of liver diseases. *Pharm Biol*. 2011. May 19. [Epub ahead of print].

Kubota Y, Iso H, Date C, et. al. Dietary Intakes of Antioxidant Vitamins and Mortality From Cardiovascular Disease: The Japan Collaborative Cohort Study (JACC) Study. *Stroke*. 2011. 42(6):1665-1672. Epub 2011 Apr 21.

409. Darvin ME, Patzelt A, Knorr F, Blume-Peytavi U, Sterry W, Lademann J. One-year study on the variation of carotenoid antioxidant substances in living human skin: influence of dietary supplementation and stress factors. *J Biomed Opt*. 2008. 13(4):044028.

410. USDA Agricultural Research Services Website. Nutrient Data Laboratory–U.S. Department of Agriculture (USDA). USDA Database for the Oxygen Radical Absorbance Capacity (ORAC) of Selected Foods, Release 2. Available at: www.ars.usda.gov/SP2UserFiles/Place/12354500/Data/ORAC/ORAC_R2.pdf. Accessed March 12, 2011.

411. Offord EA, Gautier JC, Avanti O, et al. Photoprotective potential of lycopene, beta-carotene, vitamin E, vitamin C and carnosic acid in UVA-irradiated human skin fibroblasts. *Free Radic Biol Med*. 2002. 32(12):1293-1303.

412. Beyer RE. The role of ascorbate in antioxidant protection of biomembranes: interaction with vitamin E and coenzyme Q. *J Bioenerg Biomembr*. 1994. 26(4):349-358.

Chan AC. Partners in defense, vitamin E and vitamin C. *Can J Physiol Pharmacol*. 1993. 71(9):725-731.

Stahl W, Sies H. Antioxidant defense: vitamins E and C and carotenoids. *Diabetes*. 1997. 46(Suppl 2):S14-18.

Sies H, Stahl W, Sundquist A R. Antioxidant functions of vitamins, vitamins E and C, beta-carotene, and other carotenoids. *Ann N Y Acad Sci.* 1992. 669:7–20. doi: 10.1111/j.1749-6632.1992.tb17085.x.

Stahl W, Sies H. Carotenoids and flavonoids contribute to nutritional protection against skin damage from sunlight. *Mol Biotechnol.* 2007. 37(1):26-30.

Campos PM, Gonçalves GM, Gaspar LR. In vitro antioxidant activity and in vivo efficacy of topical formulations containing vitamin C and its derivatives studied by non-invasive methods. *Skin Res Technol.* 2008. 14(3):376-380.

AOCS Lipid Library Website. Tocopherols and Tocotrienols: Structure, Composition, Biology and Analysis. Available at: http://lipidlibrary.aocs.org/lipids/tocol/index.htm. Accessed January 25, 2011.

413. Dole Website. Dole Diet Center, Glucosinolates: antioxidant fountain of youth. Available at: www.dole.com/NutritionInstituteLanding/NI_Articles/NI_DoleDiet/NI_DoleDiet_Detail/tabid/1058/Default.aspx?contentid=8930. Accessed June 13, 2011.

414. Shahidi F, Naczk M. *Phenolics in Food and Nutraceuticals.* 2nd ed. CRC Press, Boca Raton, FL. 2003.

415. Nichols JA, Katiyar SK. Skin photoprotection by natural polyphenols: anti-inflammatory, antioxidant and DNA repair mechanisms. *Arch Dermatol Res.* 2010. 302(2):71-83. Epub 2009 Nov 7.

416. Soto AM, Chung KL, Sonnenschein C. The pesticides endosulfan, toxaphene, and dieldrin have estrogenic effects on human estrogen-sensitive cells. *Environ Health Perspect.* 1994. 102(4):380-383.

417. Lee KY, Weintraub ST, Yu BP. Isolation and identification of a phenolic antioxidant from Aloe barbadensis. *Free Radi Biol Med.* 2000. 28(2):261-265.

Hu Y, Xu J, Hu Q. Evaluation of antioxidant potential of aloe vera (Aloe barbadensis miller) extracts. *J Agric Food Chem.* 2003. 51(26):7788-7791.

Hu Q, Hu Y, Xu J. Free radical-scavenging activity of Aloe vera (Aloe barbadensis miller) extracts by supercritical carbon dioxide extraction. *Food Chem.* 2005. 91(1):85-90.

Kammoun M, Miladi S, Ali YB, Damak M, Gargouri Y, Bezzine S. In vitro study of the PLA2 inhibition and antioxidant activities of Aloe vera leaf skin extracts. *Lipids Health Dis.* 2011. 10(1):14. Epub ahead of print.

ezine Articles Website. Wee J. The Truth Behind Cleopatra's Beauty. Available at: http://ezinearticles.com/?The-Truth-Behind-Cleopatras-Beauty&id=668006. Accessed March 12, 2011.

418. Markova NG, Karaman-Jurukovska N, Dong KK, Damaghi N, Smiles KA, Yarosh DB. Skin cells and tissue are capable of using L-ergothioneine as an integral component of their antioxidant defense system. *Free Radic Biol Med.* 2009. 46(8):1168-1176. Epub 2009 Feb 3.

419. World's Healthiest Foods Website. Mushrooms, shiitake. Available at: www.whfoods.com/genpage.php?tname=foodspice&dbid=122. Accessed June 13, 2011.

420. Hwang YP, Choi JH, Choi JM, Chung YC, Jeong HG. Protective mechanisms of anthocyanins from purple sweet potato against tert-butyl hydroperoxide-induced hepatotoxicity. *Food Chem Toxicol.* 2011 May 25. [Epub ahead of print].

Shahidi F, Naczk M. *Phenolics in Food and Nutraceuticals.* 2nd ed. CRC Press, Boca Raton, FL. 2003.

421. Wang L, Lu L. Pathway-specific effect of caffeine on protection against UV irradiation–induced apoptosis in corneal epithelial cells. *Invest Ophthalmol Vis Sci.* 2007. 48(2):652–660.

422. El-Salamouny S, Ranwala D, Shapiro M, Shepard BM, Farrar RR Jr. Tea, coffee, and cocoa as ultraviolet radiation protectants for the beet armyworm nucleopolyhedrovirus. *J Econ Entomol.* 2009. 102(5):1767-1773.

Wang L, Lu L. Pathway-specific effect of caffeine on protection against UV irradiation–induced apoptosis in corneal epithelial cells. *Invest Ophthalmol Vis Sci.* 2007. 48(2):652–660.

Koo SW, Hirakawa S, Fujii S, Kawasumi M, Nghiem P. Protection from photodamage by topical application of caffeine after ultraviolet irradiation. *Br J Dermatol.* 2007. 156(5):957-964. Epub 2007 Mar 28.

Conney AH, Kramata P, Lou YR, Lu YP. Effect of caffeine on UVB-induced carcinogenesis, apoptosis, and the elimination of UVB-induced patches of p53 mutant epidermal cells in SKH-1 mice. *Photochem Photobiol.* 2008. 84(2):330-338. Epub 2008 Jan 7.

423. Science Daily Website. Sunscreen in a pill: dermatologists discover sun protection under the sea. Available at: www.sciencedaily.com/videos/2007/1108-sunscreen_in_a_pill.htm. Accessed June 13, 2011.

424. Live Strong Website. Food Sources of Astaxanthin. Available at: www.livestrong.com/article/40341-sources-astaxanthin/. Accessed June 13, 2011.

Astaxanthin Growers' Association Website. Astaxanthin. Available at: www.astaxanthin.org/. Accessed December 21, 2010.

425. Kang JH. Protective effects of carnosine and homocarnosine on ferritin and hydrogen peroxide-mediated DNA damage. *BMB Rep.* 2010. 43(10):683-687.

Anti-aging Today Website. Carnosine. Available at: www.anti-aging-today.org/medicine/anti-aging/carnosine.htm. Accessed June 13, 2011.

Ozdoğan K, Taşkın E, Dursun N. Protective effect of carnosine on adriamycin-induced oxidative heart damage in rats. *Anadolu Kardiyol Derg.* 2011. 11(1):3-10. Epub 2010 Dec 24. doi: 10.5152/akd.2011.003.

426. Hipkiss A. Carnosine, diabetes, and Alzheimer's disease. *Expert Rev Neurother.* 2009. 9(5):583-585.

McFarland GA, Holliday R. Retardation of the senescence of cultured human diploid fibroblasts by carnosine. *Exp Cell Res.* 1994. 212(2):167-175.

427. Babizhayev MA. New concept in nutrition for the maintenance of the aging eye redox regulation and therapeutic treatment of cataract disease; synergism of natural antioxidant imidazole-containing amino acid-based compounds, chaperone, and glutathione boosting agents: a systemic perspective on aging and longevity emerged from studies in humans. *Am J Ther.* 2010. 17(4):373-389.

Boldyrev AA, Stvolinsky SL, Fedorova TN, Suslina ZA. Carnosine as a natural antioxidant and geroprotector: from molecular mechanisms to clinical trials. *Rejuvenation Res.* 2010. 13(2-3):156-158.

428. eHow Website. Carnosine Diet. Available at: www.ehow.com/way_5715016_carnosine-diet.html. Accessed May 4, 2011.

429. eZine Articles Website. Scott K. Alzheimer's – Rosemary, Carnosic Acid to the Rescue with a Gentla "PAT" on the Brain. Available at: http://ezinearticles.com/?Alzheimers---Rosemary,-Carnosic-Acid-To-The-Rescue-With-A-Gentle-PAT-On-The-Brain&id=854915. Accessed June 19, 2011.

Masuda T, Inaba Y, Takeda Y. Antioxidant mechanism of carnosic acid: structural identification of two oxidation products. *J Agric Food Chem.* 2001. 49(11):5560-5565.

Costa S, Utan A, Speroni E, et. al. Carnosic acid from rosemary extracts: a potential chemoprotective agent against aflatoxin B1. An in vitro study. *J App Toxicol.* 2007. 27(2):152-159.

430. Graf E. Antioxidant potential of ferulic acid. *Free Radic Biol Med.* 1992. 13(4):435-448.

Srinivasan M, Sudheer AR, Menon VP. Ferulic Acid: therapeutic potential through its antioxidant property. *J Clin Biochem Nutr.* 2007. 40(2):92-100. Available at: www.ncbi.nlm.nih.gov/pmc/articles/PMC2127228/.

Yan JJ, Cho JY, Kim HS, et al. Protection against beta-amyloid peptide toxicity in vivo with long-term administration of ferulic acid. *Br J Pharmacol.* 2001. 133(1):89-96.

431. Phytochemicals Website. Ferulic Acid. Available at: www.phytochemicals.info/phytochemicals/ferulic-acid.php. Accessed June 13, 2011.

432. Laokuldilok T, Shoemaker CF, Jongkaewwattana S, Tulyathan V. Antioxidants and antioxidant activity of several pigmented rice brans. *J Agric Food Chem.* 2011. 59(1):193-199. Epub 2010 Dec 9.

Unnamalai Agro Website. History of Vegetable Oil. Available at: http://unnamalai.net/history.php. Accessed June 19, 2011.

433. WebMD Website. Find a Vitamin or Supplement: Gama Oryzanol Overview Information. Available at: www.webmd.com/vitamins-supplements/ingredientmono-770-GAMMA+ORYZANOL.aspx?activeIngredientId=770&activeIngredientName=GAMMA+ORYZANOL. Accessed June 13, 2011.

434. Health-Care-Clinic Website. Gamma Oryzanol. Available at: www.health-care-clinic.org/alternative-medicines/gamma-oryzanol.html. Accessed June 13, 2011.

435. Moreira PI, Sayre LM, Zhu X, Nunomura A, Smith MA, Perry G. Detection and localization of markers of oxidative stress by in situ methods: application in the study of Alzheimer disease. *Methods Mol Biol.* 2010. 610:419-434.

Suite 101 Website. Burnham K. Glutathione, Turmeric, Selenium: Nutrition for Cataracts and Alzheimer's Disease. Available at: www.suite101.com/content/glutathione-turmeric-selenium-a16493. Accessed June 13, 2011.

436. Glutathione Disease Cure Website. Alzheimer's Glutathione. Available at: www.glutathionediseasecure.com/alzheimers-glutathione.html. Accessed June 13, 2011.

Suite 101 Website. Burnham K. Glutathione, Turmeric, Selenium: Nutrition for Cataracts and Alzheimer's Disease. Available at: www.suite101.com/content/glutathione-turmeric-selenium-a16493. Accessed June 13, 2011.

437. Suite 101 Website. Burnham K. Glutathione, Turmeric, Selenium: Nutrition for Cataracts and Alzheimer's Disease. Available at: www.suite101.com/content/glutathione-turmeric-selenium-a16493. Accessed June 13, 2011.

438. Vicentini FT, Fonseca YM, Pitol DL, Iyomasa MM, Bentley MV, Fonseca MJ. Evaluation of protective effect of a water-in-oil microemulsion incorporating quercetin against UVB-induced damage in hairless mice skin. *J Pharm Pharm Sci.* 2010. 13(2):274-285.

439. FRS Website. Quercetin Rich Foods. Available at: http://healthfitness.frs.com/quercetin-rich-foods-6926.html. Accessed June 13, 2011.

440. Liu Y, Chan F, Sun H, et al. Resveratrol protects human keratinocytes HaCaT cells from UVA-induced oxidative stress damage by downregulating Keap1 expression. *Eur J Pharmacol*. 2010. 650(1):130-137. Epub 2010 Oct 14.

441. Oregon State University Website. Higdon J. Resveratrol. Available at: http://lpi. oregonstate.edu/infocenter/phytochemicals/resveratrol/ .Accessed June 13, 2011.

442. Pliego K, Eastmond DA, Lovatt C. Genotoxicity and cytotoxicity testing in a human cell line for the evaluation of the antioxidant benefits of 'Hass'Avocado. SP003 In: Abstract Book: SETAC North America 30th Annual Meeting, 2010, New Orleans, LA. Available at: http://neworleans. setac.org/sites/default/files/abstract%20book.pdf. Accessed June 13, 2011.

443. Zhang Y, Talalay P, Cho CG, Posner GH. A major inducer of anticarcinogenic protective enzymes from broccoli: isolation and elucidation of structure. *Proc Natl Acad Sci USA*. 1992. 89(6):2399- 2403.

Dinkova-Kostova AT, Fahey JW, Benedict AL, et. al. Dietary glucoraphanin-rich broccoli sprout extracts protect against UV radiation-induced skin carcinogenesis in SKH-1 hairless mice. *Photochem Photobiol Sci*. 2010. 9(4):597–560.

Dinkova-Kostova AT, Jenkins SN, Fahey JW, et al. Protection against UV-light-induced skin carcinogenesis in SKH-1 high-risk mice by sulforaphane-containing broccoli sprout extracts. *Cancer Lett*. 2006. 240(2):243–252. Epub 2005 Nov 3.

Kensler TW, Chen JG, Egner PA, et al. Effects of glucosinolate-rich broccoli sprouts on urinary levels of aflatoxin-DNA adducts and phenanthrene tetraols in a randomized clinical trial in He Zuo township, Qidong, People's Republic of China. *Cancer Epidemiol Biomarkers Prev*. 2005. 14(11 Pt 1):2605-2613.

444. Life Extension Website. Coleman J. Boosting your body's store of the enzyme SOD provides powerful protection against oxidative stress. Available at: www.lef.org/magazine/mag2005/aug2005_report_sod_02.htm. Accessed June 19, 2011.

445. Reeve VE, Allanson M, Arun SJ, Domanski D, Painter N. Mice drinking goji berry juice (Lycium barbarum) are protected from UV radiation-induced skin damage via antioxidant pathways. *Photochem Photobiol Sci*. 2010. 9(4):601-607.

446. Katiyar S, Elmets CA, Katiyar SK. Green tea and skin cancer: photoimmunology, angiogenesis and DNA repair. *J Nutri Biochem*. 2007. 18(5):287-296. Epub 2006 Oct 17.

Katiyar SK. Green tea prevents non-melanoma skin cancer by enhancing DNA repair. *Arch Biochem Biophys*. 2011. 508(2):152-158. Epub 2010 Nov 19.

Katiyar S, Vaid M, van Steeg H, Meeran SM. Green tea polyphenols prevent UV-induced immunosuppression by rapid repair of DNA damage and enhancement of nucleotide excision repair genes. *Cancer Prev Res* (Phila). 2010. 3(2):179-189. Epub 2010 Jan 26.

Bouzari N, Romagosa Y, Kirsner RS. Green tea prevents skin cancer by two mechanisms. *J Invest Dermatol*. 2009. 129(5):1054.

Meeran SM, Akhtar S, Katiyar SK. Inhibition of UVB-induced skin tumor development by drinking green tea polyphenols is mediated through DNA repair and subsequent inhibition of inflammation. *J Invest Dermatol*. 2009. 129(5):1258-70. Epub 2008 Nov 20.

447. Fu YC, Jin XP, Wei SM, Lin HF, Kacew S. Ultraviolet radiation and reactive oxygen generation as inducers of keratinocyte apoptosis: protective role of tea polyphenols. *J Toxicol Environ Health A.* 2000. 61(3):177-188.

448. USDA Agricultural Research Services Website. Nutrient Data Laboratory–U.S. Department of Agriculture (USDA). USDA Database for the Oxygen Radical Absorbance Capacity (ORAC) of Selected Foods, Release 2. Available at: www.ars.usda.gov/SP2UserFiles/Place/12354500/Data/ORAC/ORAC_R2.pdf. Accessed March 12, 2011.

449. Cho S, Shin MH, Kim YK, et al. Effects of infrared radiation and heat on human skin aging in vivo. *J Investig Dermatol Symp Proc.* 2009. 14(1):15-19. doi:10.1038/jidsymp.2009.7.

   Schroeder P, Lademann J, Darvin ME, et al. Infrared radiation-induced matrix metalloproteinase in human skin: implications for protection. *J Invest Dermatol.* 2008. 128(10): 2491–2497. Epub 2008 May 1.

   Schroeder P, Krutmann J. What is needed for a sunscreen to provide complete protection. *Skin Therapy Lett.* 2010. 15(4):4-5. Available at: www.skintherapyletter.com/2010/15.4/2.html. Accessed March 19, 2011.

   Chen Z, Seo JY, Kim YK, et al. Heat modulation of tropoelastin, fibrillin-1, and matrix metalloproteinase-12 in human skin in vivo. *J Invest Dermatol.* 2005. 124(1):70-78.

450. Rass K, Reichrath J. UV damage and DNA repair in malignant melanoma and nonmelanoma skin cancer. *Adv Exp Med Biol.* 2008. 624:162-178.

451. Moison RM, Beijersbergen Van Henegouwen GM. Dietary eicosapentaenoic acid prevents systemic immunosuppression in mice induced by UVB radiation. *Radiat Res.* 2001. 156(1):36–44.

452. Black HS, Thornby JI, Gerguis J, Lenger W. Influence of dietary omega-6, -3 fatty acid sources on the initiation and promotion stages of photocarcinogenesis. *Photochem Photobiol.* 1992. 56(2):195–199.

   Cario-Andre M, Briganti S, Picardo M, Nikaido O, de Verneuil H, Taieb A. Polyunsaturated fatty acids partially reproduce the role of melanocytes in the epidermal melanin unit. *Exp Dermatol.* 2005. 14(3):194–201.

   Black HS, Rhodes LE. The potential of omega-3 fatty acids in the prevention of non-melanoma skin cancer. *Cancer Detect Prev.* 2006. 30(3):224-232. Epub 2006 Jul 26.

453. Hakim IA, Harris RB, Ritenbaugh C. Fat intake and risk of squamous cell carcinoma of the skin. *Nutr Cancer.* 2000. 36(2):155–162.

   McCusker MM, Grant-Kels JM. Healing fats of the skin: the structural and immunologic roles of the omega-6 and omega-3 fatty acids. *Clin Dermatol.* 2010. 28(4):440-451.

454. Antoniou C, Kosmadaki MG, Stratigos AJ, Katsambas AD. Photoaging: prevention and topical treatments. *Am J Clin Dermatol.* 2010. 11(2):95-102. doi: 10.2165/11530210-000000000-00000.

455. Viola P, Viola M. Virgin olive oil as a fundamental nutritional component and skin protector. *Clin Dermatol.* 2009. 27(2):159-165.

   Willett WC. The Mediterranean diet: science and practice. *Public Health Nutr.* 2006. 9(1A):105-110.

456. Omar SH. Oleuropein in olive and its pharmacological effects. *Sci Pharm.* 2010. 78(2):133-154.

457. Omar SH. Oleuropein in olive and its pharmacological effects. *Sci Pharm.* 2010. 78(2):133-154.

Budiyanto A, Ahmed NU, Wu A, et. al. Protective effect of topically applied olive oil against photocarcinogenesis following UVB exposure of mice. *Carcinogenesis*. 2000. 21(11):2085-2090.

Kimura Y, Sumiyoshi M. Olive leaf extract and its main component oleuropein prevent chronic ultraviolet B radiation-induced skin damage and carcinogenesis in hairless mice. *J Nutr*. 2009. 139: 2079–2086. Epub 2009 Sep 23.

458. Camouse MM, Domingo DS, Swain FR, et al. Topical application of green and white tea extracts provides protection from solar-simulated ultraviolet light in human skin. *Exp Dermatol*. 2009. 18(6):522-526.

459. Katiyar S, Elmets CA, Katiyar SK. Green tea and skin cancer: photoimmunology, angiogenesis and DNA repair. J NutriBiochem. 2007. 18(5):287-296. Epub 2006 Oct 17.

460. Schroeder P, Lademann J, Darvin ME, Stege H, Marks C, Bruhnke S, Krutmann J. Infrared radiation-induced matrix metalloproteinase in human skin: implications for protection. *J Invest Dermatol*. 2008. 128(10):2491-2497. Epub 2008 May 1.

461. Life Extension Website. Coleman J. Boosting your body's store of the enzyme SOD provides powerful protection against oxidative stress. Available at: www.lef.org/magazine/mag2005/aug2005_report_sod_02.htm. Accessed June 19, 2011.

462. Stahl W, Sies H. Carotenoids and flavonoids contribute to nutritional protection against skin damage from sunlight. *Mol Biotechnol*. 2007. 37(1):26-30.

463. Kansas Historical Society Website. Cool Things: Bathing Suit. Available at: www.kshs.org/p/cool-things-bathing-suit/10297. Accessed January 18, 2011.

Coronado History Website: Bathing Suits. Available at: www.coronadohistory.org/Store/popup_pb1.html. Accessed January 18, 2011.

464. Alibaba Website. UV-cut Fabric. Available at: www.alibaba.com/product-free/104030826/UV_CUT_fabric.html. Accessed June 13, 2011.

UPF Apparel Website. UPF Rating System. Available at: www.upfapparel.com/UPFRatings. Accessed June 13, 2011.

465. Gambichler T, Hatch KL, Avermaete A, et al. Ultraviolet protection factor of fabrics: comparison of laboratory and field-based measurements. *Photodermatol Photoimmunol Photomed*. 2002. 18(3):135-140.

466. Gambichler T, Altmeyer P, Hoffmann K. Comparison of methods: determination of UV protection of clothing. *Recent Results Cancer Res*. 2002;160:55-61.

467. Sunshine Products Website. Common Questions and Answers about SunSoul Products. Available at: www.sunscreenwear.com/technology/faq.html. Accessed January 6, 2011.

468. Vigneshwaran N, Kumar S, Kathe AA, Varadarajan PV, Prasad V. Functional finishing of cotton fabrics using zinc oxide–soluble starch nanocomposites. Nanotechnology. 2006. 17(20):5087-5095. doi: 10.1088/0957-4484/17/20/008.

469. Made-in-China Website. Nano Titanium Dioxide for Fabric (ZXL-001). Available at: www.made-in-china.com/showroom/laiyangzixilai/product-detailqMKxcyDPCaRo/China-Nano-Titanium-Dioxide-for-Fabric-ZXL-001-.html. Accessed June 13, 2011.

470. Technology Review (MIT) Website. Patel P. Clothes that clean themselves: Australian researchers are developing a process that could lead to self-cleaning wool sweaters and silk ties. Available at: www.technologyreview.com/Nanotech/20306/?a=f#comment-220396. Accessed March 13, 2011.

Kuno Y. *Human Perspiration*. CC Thomas. Springfield, Il. 1956. Cited in *The Apocrine Glands and the Breast*. Craigmyle M, Buchanan L. John Wiley and Sons. 1984. Page 16.

471. Rajendran R, Balakumar C, Hasabo A, et al. Use of zinc oxide nano particles for production of antimicrobial textiles. *Int J Eng Sci Technol*. 2010. 2(1):202-208.

472. Fibre 2 Fashion Website. Das S. Some important facts of titanium dioxide used in textile industry – a challenge to nanotechnology. Available at: www. fibre2fashion.com/industry-article/1/71/some-important-facts-of-titanium-dioxide-used-in-textile-industry1.asp. Accessed January 26, 2011.

473. Richardson BA. Sudden infant death syndrome: a possible primary cause. *J Forensic Sci Soc*. 1994. 34(3):199-204.

Fleming PJ, Cooke M, Chantler SM, Golding J. Fire retardants, biocides, plasticisers, and sudden infant deaths. *BMJ*. 1994. 309(6969):1594-1596.

474. Chen D, Hale RC. A global review of polybrominated diphenyl ether flame retardant contamination in birds. *Environ Int*. 2010. 36(7):800-811. Epub 2010 Jun 16.

475. Rudel RA, Dodson RE, Perovich LJ, et al. Semivolatile endocrine-disrupting compounds in paired indoor and outdoor air in two northern California communities. *Environ Sci Technol*. 2010. 44(17):6583-6590.

Zota AR, Rudel RA, Morello-Frosch RA, Brody JG. Elevated house dust and serum concentrations of PBDEs in California: Unintended consequences of furniture flammability standards. *Environ. Sci. Technol*. 2008. 42(12):8158–8164.

476. Herbstman JB, Sjödin A, Kurzon M, et al. Prenatal exposure to PBDEs and neurodevelopment. *Environ Health Perspect*. 2010. 118(5):712-719. Epub 2010 Jan 4.

Chemical & Engineering News Website. Betts K. Children's Blood Containing High Levels of PBDE Fire Retardants. Available at: www.pubs.acs.org/cen/news/88/i26/8826news1.html. Accessed June 20, 2011.

477. Chemical & Engineering News Website. Hess G. House Opens Inquiry into Fire Retardants. Available at: www.pubs.acs.org/cen/environment/88/8816govc2. html. Accessed January 26, 2011.

478. Shaw SD, Blum A, Weber R, et al. Halogenated flame retardants: do the fire safety benefits justify the risks? *Rev Environ Health*. 2010. 25(4):261-305.

479. Beasley DG, Meyer TA. Characterization of the UVA protection provided by avobenzone, zinc oxide, and titanium dioxide in broad-spectrum sunscreen products. Am J Clin Dermatol. 2010. 11(6):413-421.

480. Chatelain E, Gabard B. Photostabilization of butyl methoxydibenzoylmethane (Avobenzone) and ethylhexyl methoxycinnamate by bis-ethylhexyloxyphenol methoxyphenyl triazine (Tinosorb S), a new UV broadband filter. *Photochem Photobiol*. 2001. 74(3):401-406.

481. Fourtanir A, Moyal D, Seite S. Sunscreens containing the broad-spectrum UVA absorber, Mexoryl SX, prevent the cutaneous detrimental effects of UV exposure: a review of clinical study results. *Photodermatol Photoimmunol Photomed*. 2008. 24(4):164–174.

482. Schroeder P, Krutmann J. What is needed for a sunscreen to provide complete protection. Skin Therapy Lett. 2010. 15(4):4-5. Available at: www. skintherapyletter.com/2010/15.4/2.html.

483. Vettor M, Bourgeois S, Fessi H, et al. Skin absorption studies of octyl-methoxycinnamate loaded poly(D,L-lactide) nanoparticles: estimation of the UV filter distribution and release behaviour in skin layers. *J Microencapsul*. 2010. 27(3):253-262.

Jiménez MM, Pelletier J, Bobin MF, Martini MC. Influence of encapsulation on the in vitro percutaneous absorption of octyl methoxycinnamate. *Int J Pharm*. 2004. 272(1-2):45-55.

Golmohammadzadeh S, Jaafarixx MR, Khalili N. Evaluation of liposomal and conventional formulations of octyl methoxycinnamate on human percutaneous absorption using the stripping method. *J Cosmet Sci*. 2008. 59(5):385-398.

Wolf P, Cox P, Yarosh DB, Kripke ML. Sunscreens and T4N5 liposomes differ in their ability to protect against ultraviolet-induced sunburn cell formation, alterations of dendritic epidermal cells, and local suppression of contact hypersensitivity. *J Invest Dermatol*. 1995. 104(2):287–292.

484. Scalia S, Coppi G, Iannuccelli V. Microencapsulation of a cyclodextrin complex of the UV filter, butyl methoxydibenzoylmethane: in vivo skin penetration studies. *J Pharm Biomed Anal*. 2011. 54(2):345-350. Epub 2010 Sep 19.

485. Abdel-Malek ZA, Kadekaro AL, Swope VB. Stepping up melanocytes to the challenge of UV Exposure. *Pigment Cell Melanoma Res*. 2010. 23(2):171–186. Epub 2010 Feb 1.

486. eMedicine Website. Amirlak B. Skin anatomy. Available at: http://emedicine. medscape.com/article/1294744-overview#aw2aab6b3. Accessed June 13, 2010.

487. Clinuvel Website. Function of skin pigment. Available at: www.clinuvel.com/ dermatology/melanin/function-skin-pigment. Accessed June 19, 2011.

Becker SW. Melanin Pigmentation. Arch Derm Syphilol. 1927. 16(3):259-290.

488. Yarosh D, Klein J, O'Connor A, Hawk J, Rafal E, Wolf P. Effect of topically applied T4 endonuclease V in liposomes on skin cancer in xeroderma pigmentosum: a randomised study. Xeroderma Pigmentosum Study Group. *Lancet*. 2001. 357(9260): 926–929.

Antoniou C, Kosmadak MG, Stratigos AJ, Katsambas AD. Sunscreens – what's important to know. *J Eur Acad Derm Venereol*. 2008. 22(9):1110–1119. Epub 2008 Aug 18. DOI: 10.1111/j.1468-3083.2007.02580.x.

489. Balskus EP, Walsh CT. The genetic and molecular basis for sunscreen biosynthesis in cyanobacteria. *Science*. 2010. 329(5999):1653-1656. Epub 2010 Sept 2.

490. Antoniou C, Kosmadaki MG, Stratigos AJ, Katsambas AD. Photoaging: prevention and topical treatments. *Am J Clin Dermatol*. 2010. 11(2):95-102. doi: 10.2165/11530210-000000000-00000.

491. Dong KK, Damaghi N, Picart SD, et al. UV-induced DNA damage initiates release of MMP-1 in human skin. *Exp Dermatol*. 2008. 17(12):1037-1044. Epub 2008 May 3.

492. Abdel-Malek ZA, Kadekaro AL, Swope VB. Stepping up melanocytes to the challenge of UV Exposure. *Pigment Cell Melanoma Res*. 2010. 23(2):171–186. Epub 2010 Feb 1.

493. Oresajo C, Yatskayer M, Galdi A, Foltis P, Pillai S. Complementary effects of antioxidants and sunscreens in reducing UV-induced skin damage as demonstrated by skin biomarker expression. *J Cosmet Laser Ther*. 2010. 12(3):157–162.

International Centre for Science and High Technology Website. Medicinal and aromatic plants: Senna alta (L.) Roxb. Available at: http://portal.ics.trieste. it/maps/MedicinalPlants_Plant.aspx?id=654. Accessed June 12, 2011.

494. Gilaberte Y, González S. Update on photoprotection. *Actas Dermosifiliogr*. 2010. 101(8):659-672.

Schroeder P, Krutmann J. What is needed for a sunscreen to provide complete protection. *Skin Therapy Lett.* 2010. 15(4):4-5. Available at: www.skintherapyletter.com/2010/15.4/2.html.

495. Abdel-Malek ZA, Kadekaro AL, Swope VB. Stepping up melanocytes to the challenge of UV Exposure. *Pigment Cell Melanoma Res.* 2010. 23(2):171–186. Epub 2010 Feb 1.

496. Schroeder P, Krutmann J. What is needed for a sunscreen to provide complete protection. *Skin Therapy Lett.* 2010. 15(4):4-5. Available at: www.skintherapyletter.com/2010/15.4/2.html.

497. Otto A, du Plessis J, Wiechers JW. Formulation effects of topical emulsions on transdermal and dermal delivery. *Int J Cosmet Sci.* 2009. 31(1):1-19.

498. Rivers JK. The role of cosmeceuticals in antiaging therapy. Skin Therapy Lett. 2008. 13(8):5-9.

499. Bissonnette, R. Update on sunscreens. *Skin Therapy Lett.* 2008. 13(6):5-7. Available at: www.medscape.com/viewarticle/582990. Accessed June 12, 2011.

500. Cancer News in Context Website. Does Sunscreen Prevent Skin Cancers? Available at: www.cancernewsincontext.org/2010/07/does-sunscreen-prevent-skin-cancer.html. Accessed January 2, 2011.

Marks R. The changing incidence and mortality of melanoma in Australia. *Recent Results Cancer Res.* 2002. 160:113-121.

501. Australian Government: Therapeutic Goods Admin (TGA) Website. Consultation: Australian Regulatory Guidelines for OTC Medicines – Sunscreens. Available at: www.tga.gov.au/npmeds/consult/cons-argom-sunscreens.htm. Document available at: www.tga.gov.au/npmeds/consult/cons-argom-sunscreens.pdf. Accessed January 26, 2011.

502. Faurschou A, Wulf HC. Ecological analysis of the relation between sunbeds and skin cancer. Photodermatol Photoimmunol Photomed. 2007. 23(4):120-125.

503. Armas LA, Fusaro RM, Sayre RM, Huerter CJ, Heaney RP. Do melanoidins induced by topical 9% dihydroxyacetone sunless tanning spray inhibit vitamin d production? A pilot study. *Photochem Photobiol.* 2009. 85(5):1265-1266. Epub 2009 May 28.

504. CDC Website. Ansdell VE. Sunburn. Available at: wwwnc.cdc.gov/travel/yellowbook/2010/chapter-2/sunburn.aspx. Accessed January 24, 2011.

505. Science Daily Website. Nanoparticles Used in Common Household Items Cause Genetic Damage in Mice. Available at: www.sciencedaily.com/releases/2009/11/091116165739.htm. Accessed February 10, 2011. Interview of co-author of: Trouiller B, Reliene R, Westbrook A, Solaimani P, Schiestl RH. Titanium dioxide nanoparticles induce DNA damage and genetic instability in vivo in mice. Cancer Res. 2009. 69(22):8784-8789. Epub 2009 Nov 3.

506. Matts PJ, Fink B. Chronic sun damage and the perception of age, health and attractiveness. Photochem. Photobiol. Sci. 2010. 9(4):421–431.

507. Hertog MGL, Hollman PCH, Katan MB. Content of potentially anticarcinogenic flavonoids of 28 vegetables and 9 fruits commonly consumed in the Netherlands. J Agric Food Chem.1992. 40(12):2379-2383. DOI:10.1021/jf00024a011.

Rousseff RL, Martin SF, Youtsey CO. Quantitative survey of narirutin, naringin, heperidin, and neohesperidin in Citrus. J Agric Food Chem. 1987. 35:1027-1030.

Clifford MN. Anthocyanins in foods. 1996 Symposium on polyphenols and anthocyanins as food colourants and antioxidants, Brussels, Belgium, EU. 1996. Pages 1–19.

Tsushida T, Svzuki M. Content of flavonol glucosides and some properties of enzymes metabolizing the glucosides in onion. 3. Flavonoid in fruits and vegetables. J Jpn Soc Food Sci Technol. 1996. 43:642–649.

Hertog MG, Hollman PCH, van de Putte B. Content of potentially anticarcinogenic flavonoids of tea infusions, wine and fruit juices. J Agric Food Chem. 1993. 41(8):1242-1246.

Burda S, Oleszek W, Lee CY. Phenolic compounds and their changes in apples during maturation and cold storage. J Agric Food Chem. 1990. 38(4):945-948.

Santos-Buelga C, Scalbert A. Proanthocyanidins and tannin-like compounds – nature, occurrence, dietary intake and effects on nutrition and health. J Sci Food Agric. 2000. 80(7):1094-1117. doi: 10.1002/(SICI)1097-0010(20000515)80:7<1094::AID-JSFA569>3.0.CO;2-1

Kroon PA, Faulds CB, Ryden P, Robertson JA, Williamson G. (1997). Release of covalently bound ferulic acid from fiber in the human colon. J Agric Food Chem. 1997. 45(3):661-667.

Clifford MN. Chlorogenic acids and other cinnamates: nature, occurrence and dietary burden. J Sci Food Agric. 1999. 79(3):362-372.

Axelson M, Sjovall J, Gustafsson BE, Setchell KD. Origin of lignans in mammals and identification of a precursor from plants. Nature. 1982. 298(5875):659-660.

Scalbert A, Williamson G. Dietary intake and bioavailability of polyphenols. J Nutr. 2000. 130(8S suppl):2073S-2085S.

508. Scientific Committee on Consumer Products (SCCP) OPINION ON 4-Methylbenzylidene camphor (4-MBC) available at: http://ec.europa.eu/health/ph_risk/co508mmittees/04_sccp/docs/sccp_o_141.pdf. Accessed June 19, 2011.

Index

genotoxicity, 115, 121, 132
global temperature, 108, 114
 ocean temperature, 107-113,
 139
glucosinolates, 182, 193
glutathione, 131, 188-192
gynecomastia (male breast enlargement), 92-93

H

hair follicles, 7, 124
Health Council of the Netherlands,
 175
Heaney, Robert, 170
herbivores, 109
histadine, 178, 184, 187
Holick, Michael, 170
human fetus, 39, 47, 75-76, 78,
 83, 86, 88, 94, 99-100, 102-
 103, 106, 137, 142
hyperactivity disorder (adhd),
 102-103
hypodermis, 6-7, 22, 25, 144-145
hypospadias, 76, 84-90
 incidence rate, 76, 86-88, 90
hypothalamo-pituitary-gonadal
 system, 54, 80, 98

I

immune system, 27, 138, 186,
 196, 222
immunosuppression, 37, 194, 198
incidence rates

autism, 99-100, 102
basal cell carcinoma, 13-14
cancers, 11, 88, 94, 156
cryptorchidism, 85-86, 90
male reproductive organ dysgenesis, 76, 84, 88-89
melanoma, 9-14, 217
skin cancers, 9, 14, 27, 33, 62,
 143, 156
squamous cell carcinoma, 13-14
testicular cancer, 87, 90, 156
infertility, 131
 male, 88-90
infrared (IR), 17-18, 143-150, 201
 IRA, 17-18, 144-147, 149-150,
 179
 IRB, 17, 144-145
 IRC, 17, 144-145
Internal Medicine News, 89
International Society for Developmental Origins of Health and
 Disease (DOHaD), 103
intersex fish, 62
Ireland, 36

J

Japan, 23, 93, 99, 115, 256
jasmine 4
Journal of Chromatography, 73
Journal of Clinical Oncology, 11
*Journal of Investigative Dermatol-
 ogy*, 11
*Journal of Nanoscience and Nano-
 techology*, 135

Z